*LEVER*AGING HEALTH

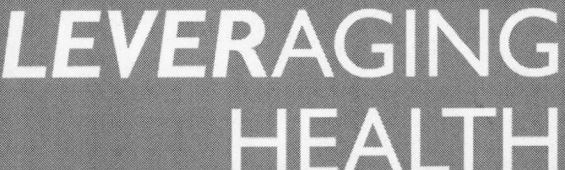

*Improve health status and bend the trend
on financial inflation with
value-based designs.*

**CYNDY NAYER, MA
JACK MAHONEY, MD
JAN BERGER, MD**

ISBN: 1-4392-4567-3
ISBN-13: 9781439245675

Visit www.booksurge.com to order additional copies.

We would like to thank the following innovators for their contributions to this book:

Ardis Belknap *
Human Resources Manager
City of Springfield, OR

Wayne N Burton, MD
Adjunct Professor of Environmental and
Occupational Health Sciences
University of Illinois at Chicago

Laura Carabello
Publisher and Managing Editor
Medical Travel Today
www.medicaltraveltoday.com

A. Mark Fendrick, MD
Professor, Internal Medicine and Health Management & Policy
Co-Director, Center for Value-Based Insurance Design
University of Michigan

Bill Germanakos
Winner, NBC Season 4 - *The Biggest Loser*
Director, Corporate Wellness
Quest Diagnostics Inc.

Peter Hayes *
Director of Associate Health and Wellness
Hannaford Supermarkets
Secretary, Center for Health Value Innovation

Bob Holben *
Director, Global Total Rewards and Int'l HR
Gulfstream Aerospace

Dave Johnson, MD, MBA, CPE *
President, Vivacity

Gregg Kamas
Director of Health Risk Management
IMA Financial Group, Inc.

Robert Kritzler, MD *
Deputy Chief Medical Officer
Johns Hopkins Health Care LLC
Vice President, Center for Health Value Innovation

Mike Kushner
Director, Risk Management
Polk County, FL

Chris McSwain *
Director, Global Benefits
Whirlpool Corporation
Vice President, Center for Health Value Innovation

Kavita V. Nair, Ph.D *
Associate Professor, School of Pharmacy University of Colorado Denver
Vice President & Treasurer, Center for Health Value Innovation

Kevin O'Brien *
CEO of Partners in Care
a physician organization in New Jersey

Thomas Parry, Ph.D.
President
Integrated Benefits Institute

Jerry Reeves, MD *
Chief Medical Officer
H.E.R.E.I.U. Welfare Funds

Robert Scully, MD *
Senior Medical Director
Health Alliance Medical Plans

Neal Sofian
Director Behavioral Interventions
Resolution Health

Brian Sweet, B.S. Pharm., M.B.A.*
Chief Pharmacy Officer
WellPoint, Inc.

Michael Taylor, MD *
Medical Director for Health Promotion Caterpillar
Chairman of the Board, Center for Health Value Innovation

Albert Tzeel, MD, MHSA *
Regional Market Medical Officer
Great Lakes Region
Humana Inc

Fred Williams*
Director, Health Management Strategies
Quest Diagnostics

Raymond J. Zastrow, MD, FAAFP *
President, QuadMed
Vice President, Center for Health Value Innovation

* Member of the Board of Directors, Center for Health Value
Innovation

FOREWORD

<u>Leveraging Health</u> is an important and very timely book for both purchasers and providers of health care. It's important to notice the wording here: it's about health. The costs of health care have gone up enormously over the past few decades while all too many outcomes have tracked in the opposite direction: more obesity, more chronic disease, more depression, and the list goes on.

The question really is about health, not health care, so perhaps we have been asking the wrong question; instead of "How much is this going to cost?" we should have been asking "How can we drive health?" or "How much of an increase in health and productivity can I expect?"

I have worked with the authors of this book for a long time. Together, we have shared insights to health and productivity management. They have fostered new paradigms in managing population health instead of disease. They have structured communications, embarked on data analysis, and educated purchasers and providers. We have, together, worked hard to change the dynamics of health and health care, focusing on the needs of our populations instead of focusing on the diseases.

We are aligned in our thinking: when we put the person at the center of our efforts, we achieve better outcomes for the person, the organization, the health plan and, especially, our communities.

So, at this time of economic crisis, with the inextricable link to health care, it's time to take bold moves. It's time to change the questions, drive for better outcomes, link productivity gains with the financial improvements, and change course. It's time for all of us to be accountable for our own health and the health of our communities. It's time to assume the leadership position once again.

<u>Leveraging Health</u> could not have appeared at a better moment in our history!

WAYNE N BURTON MD
ADJUNCT PROFESSOR OF ENVIROMENTAL AND
OCCUPATIONAL HEALTH SCIENCES
UNIVERSITY OF ILLINOIS AT CHICAGO

INTRODUCTION

This book was written for benefits decision-makers to provide a simple set of examples of innovative benefit design driven by the need to enhance every dollar spent on health in the US. With an economic impact of $2.3trillion dollars in 2008, the intersection of community health and economic security is at risk. Because of the men and women who approached the health and productivity of their workforces and their communities with a fresh set of questions, new evidence is being showcased that we hope will influence others to re-frame their intent.

In the past 25 years, cost compression has done little to slow the growth of chronic disease and related costs. Our goal here is to showcase the kinds of actions—the levers—that have delivered results to small, medium and large companies, both in the private corporate setting and in the municipal settings of cities, counties and states. Levers are a metaphor for plan designs, incentives & disincentives that cause desired behaviors.

Our work has been our passion. Our intent has been very focused—to give you a multitude of ideas to change the financial cost escalation due to poorly managed health. Our hope is that this book will provide some answers, and that you and your service providers—the health plans, broker-consultants, physician organizations and hospital systems, and everyone who provides you with guidance on health management—will join us in the movement for purchasing units of health, rather than units of healthcare.

You will, throughout this book, see case studies and quotes from some of the people who have contributed to our thinking, supported our efforts at education, and influenced their own communities. But you can be sure there were many more companies and renegades—folks who asked the questions differently and boldly implemented new strategies—who quietly contributed to our efforts.

We hope you will re-think the questions you are asking and the purchases in health that you are making. Together, we can make a difference in the lives of the people at our work, in our community, and in our country.

To your health!

Cyndy, Jack and Jan

JOHN J. MAHONEY, M.D., M.P.H.

John J. (Jack) Mahoney is retired from Pitney Bowes where, as Strategic Healthcare Initiatives Director, he was a key team leader for the company's innovative healthcare programs. Dr. Mahoney's responsibilities included advanced healthcare planning for employees and benefits planning for employees and retirees. Subsequent to retiring from his full-time position, Dr. Mahoney has assumed the role of Chief Consultant for Strategic Health Initiatives at Pitney Bowes and continues to be active in shaping the company's healthcare programs. In addition, he is the Medical Director of the Florida Healthcare Coalition.

Dr. Mahoney joined Pitney Bowes in 1997 as Corporate Medical Director and Global Healthcare Management Director. In this role he was responsible for designing health benefits for employees, and integrating disability and disease management and wellness initiatives. He also had oversight for all clinical support services.

Dr. Mahoney was instrumental in revamping the company's health insurance system in 2002. At this time, Pitney Bowes became the first company in the country to fully implement the strategy known as value-based insurance design, in which the employer uses financial incentives to encourage workers to stay healthy. Medical plan design, as well as services related to direct on-site medical care delivery, wellness, fitness, employee assistance and disability management programs are included in this integrated approach to health.

Prior to joining Pitney Bowes, Dr. Mahoney served as Vice President of Integrated Health Management at Aetna Inc., where he was responsible for integrating all health-related employee programs within Aetna to achieve improved employee productivity and effectiveness. Dr. Mahoney was also a partner with Hewitt Associates LLC, designing a wide array of managed medical benefits programs. He also served as the Corporate Medical Director for GTE Corporation and held medical management positions in the airline industry.

Dr. Mahoney received his undergraduate degree from Boston College and his Medical Degree from the Medical College of Virginia. He also received a Masters Degree in Public Health from UCLA.

Cyndy Nayer, MA

Cyndy Nayer is the President and Chief Executive Officer of the Center for Health Value Innovation, a community of employers and payers building evidence, tools and competency in value-based design for improved health and reduced cost trends. She is one of the five equal founders of the Center, along with Jack Mahoney MD, Global Health Strategy consultant for Pitney Bowes, who serves as Chief Medical Officer for the Center.

Cyndy also leads River City Partnership on Health, Inc., a national employer health strategy company linking employers, health plans, and providers in improved Total Health Management. Nayer holds a graduate degree in Gerontology with a special focus on healthy aging. As the former Chair of the Missouri Governor's Council on Health, Nayer led the call to action and strategy for the Office of Women's Health.

A futurist and health improvement expert, Cyndy was recently voted one of the emerging leaders on consumer directed health and a visionary for health transformation. She speaks and writes for national media on the concepts of consumer and employer health engagement, and she has developed worksite health strategies for Fortune 100 companies in the US and in Canada. Cyndy was awarded the CEO Leadership award in Consumer Driven Health by CDHC Solutions in September 2008. She is an honored Woman of Worth, the first recipient of the Missouri State

Health and Fitness Professional Award, a graduate of the Missouri Focus on Women's Leadership and the recipient of the American Heart Association Letter of Commendation for the Aetna Women's Health Toolkit. She has recently published a consumer handbook for value-based health decisions, entitled <u>101 Lifetips for Personal Health Management</u>.

Nayer has served as Director of Marketing for ConnectCare, the public health system in St. Louis, and she is the former Director of Health and Fitness for the St. Louis Jewish Community Center. As one of the five senior business channel directors, she developed the pharmaceutical consulting business channel for The Benfield Group. Nayer is a graduate of Washington University in St. Louis, and she holds a Masters Degree in Gerontology from Lindenwood University in St. Charles, Missouri. She is married and has two daughters.

Jan Berger, MD MJ

Jan is the founder of Health Intelligence Partners, a health-care consultancy that focuses on healthcare business strategies and solutions-based product development support in order to maximize client outcomes. Her list of clients includes large employer coalitions, business development organizations focused on medical devices, healthcare private equity companies, healthcare focused advertising agencies, large pharmaceutical manufacturers, and a peer-reviewed healthcare journal. Jan spends a large portion of her time as strategic advisor to the Center for Health Value Innovation where she works closely with Cyndy and Jack.

Prior to starting Health Intelligence Partners, Jan spent 10 years as Senior Vice President and Chief Clinical Officer for CVS Caremark (1999–2009). She has experience in healthcare policy and strategy, pharmacy benefit services, specialty pharmacy, Medicare Part D, disease and health management and health information technology. Prior to coming to CVS Caremark, Jan had 15 years' experience in healthcare administration within the health plan and academic arenas.

As Editor in Chief of American Journal of Pharmacy Benefit and on the editorial boards of a number of healthcare journals, Jan is considered a national healthcare thought leader. She speaks and writes on a broad range of healthcare issues. She also serves on numerous healthcare boards and committees and has published over 100 articles and publications.

Dr. Berger holds both a Doctor of Medicine Degree and a Masters Degree in Jurisprudence from Loyola University in Chicago and a Certificate in Healthcare Business Administration from University of South Florida. She is also an assistant professor at Northwestern University School of Medicine in Evanston, Illinois.

Chapter 1

HEALTH MANAGEMENT IN RECENT HISTORY

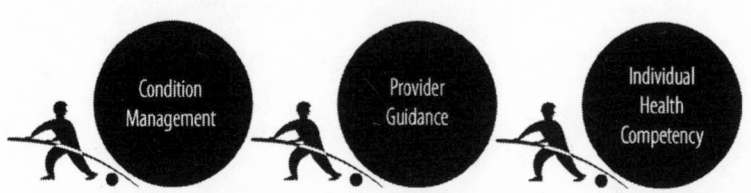

Once again, our country is examining the status of healthcare. Hard questions regarding access, quality, affordability and efficiency are being debated. Payment for care is core to this discussion, and understanding how we arrived at our current payment state gives us some insight not only into these questions, but also provides a basis for understanding the behaviors underlying health and healthcare.

These questions are not new. A recent Kaiser Family Foundation post by Drew Altman[1] itemizes the key concepts of healthcare reform that have surfaced every 19.7 years in our country's debates since the earliest health plans were put into place.

A Brief History of Health Reform

Who/When	What	Fate
Harry Truman (1950)	**Universal**	**"a socialist plot"**
LBJ (1965)	Medicare/ Medicaid	"Nothing in this Title shall be construed to authorize any Federal officer or employee to exercise any supervision or control over the practice of medicine..."
Nixon/Ford/	**Universal,**	**Mills falls in Tidal**
Wilbur Mills (1974)	**employer mandate**	**Basin with Fanne Fox**
Jimmy Carter (1979	Cost containment	The "Voluntary Effort"
Bill Clinton (1994)	**Health Security Act**	**You know the story**
Bill Clinton (1997)	S-CHIP	Number of uninsured children falls
Bill Clinton (1998)	Medicare Prescription Drug Act	Progress and privatization
Obama & Congress (2008)	**?**	**?**

Average time between major national health reform windows: 19.7 years

Source: Kaiser Family Foundation

The concept of health "insurance" first emerged during the Depression. Anxious to find ways of covering uncompensated care, hospitals collaborated in the creation of insurance specifically for hospitalizations through "Blue Cross." This expanded to coverage of physicians' services through "Blue Shield." The financial burden for these insurance vehicles was largely, if not entirely, borne by individuals. For a variety of reasons, including cost, much of the medical care given at that time was reactive. Patients accessed care for a symptomatic medical problem, beginning with a physician office visit and perhaps, followed by a hospital stay. A key element of this approach was coverage for catastrophic care.

There was little focus on preventive care or chronic condition management.

The financial constraints existing during WWII provided the impetus for moving financial responsibility for healthcare coverage from the individual to employers. This change in payment model set the stage for fundamental changes in the responsibilities of the patient, physician and employer (payer). Providers, anxious to implement the multitude of new advances and technology, complete with the hope of new health and vitality, raised their charges. Patients (the consumers) were largely isolated from financial decisions; that responsibility shifted to the plan sponsor or employer. This dynamic was further heightened with the advent of Medicare and Medicaid and the role of government in a sustainable safety net of healthcare. This "security of coverage" began to permeate most insurance discussions throughout the next 20 years.

The 1970's saw an increase in medical costs that concerned both the government and employers. The payers of healthcare insurance looked to find a new model that would stem the healthcare cost trends.

Thought leaders within healthcare believed that if there was greater focus and a more proactive role in the prevention of illness, costs could be controlled. Catastrophic care continued to be covered as in the previous model, but health plans also began to cover care to manage rising costs and control trends. In order to do so, well-person check-ups, preventive screenings and immunizations were provided with only a nominal out-of-pocket cost to the patient. As the coverage rules changed, the patient and physician conversations regarding cost of these services continued to decrease and eventually did not occur at all. In fact, rarely did patients or their physician know the costs of the care that was given.

During this time, coverage for medications also began the transfer from the patient to the plan sponsor (typically the employer-payer), and it was not unusual to see out-of-pocket co-pays in the $2 - $5 range. These low costs were associated with the desire from the payers and plans for patients to take advantage of these healthcare services in order to control unnecessary use of emergency department and inpatient days.

Along with these financial changes came quality programs and initiatives that focused on some of these previously uncovered preventive healthcare activities, such as annual check-ups for adults, regular/well anticipatory check-ups for children, and immunizations for persons of all ages. It was recognized by the insurers, employers and quality organizations, such as the National Committee for Quality Assurance, that these care activities could help to keep people healthy and control some of the healthcare costs that were burdening payers and patients.

Not only were quality organizations looking at care for the well as a financial and quality issue, they also began looking at the care that patients with chronic illness were receiving. They found that the increasing prevalence of chronic health conditions was contributing to the increasing healthcare costs. Reviews of patient records and administrative data found that many persons with these conditions were not receiving quality care necessary to improve their health and to simultaneously contain the significant healthcare costs often associated with these chronic conditions.

This increased focus on access and quality stifled the health cost trends for a period of time, but by the late 1990s, once again, healthcare costs were increasing. In response to the escalating burden of healthcare costs to the payers, increasing cost-share was once again transferred to the patient. This growing financial burden on patients became a barrier to the very services that payers wanted patients to utilize.

Today, there are reform movements on Capitol Hill, in every state legislature, at the city and county levels, as well as in community advocacy groups and living rooms throughout the United States. What will reform bring? What should it do? And who will pay for it?

1.1 Today's Environment:

The Economics of Healthcare from the Employer Perspective

Fast forward to the realities of today where employers and the private sector pay approximately 54% of the total cost of healthcare[2] and healthcare costs are increasing at an unsustainable rate. The Kaiser Family Foundation frames its study with the following facts:

- In 2007, the U.S. spent $2.2 trillion on healthcare, an average of $7,421 per person.

- The share of economic activity (gross domestic product, or GDP) devoted to healthcare has increased from 7.2 percent in 1970 to 16.2 percent in 2007.

- Healthcare costs have grown on average 2.4 percentage points faster than the GDP since 1970.

- Almost half of healthcare spending is used to treat just 5 percent of the population.[3]

The following graph shows where the health dollars are spent in America.

Distribution of National Health Expenditures by Type of Service, 2007

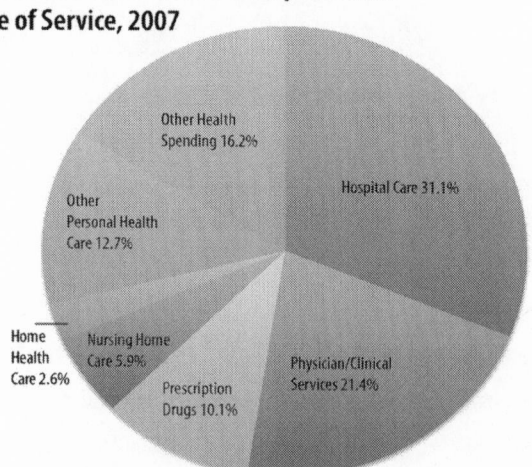

"Other Personal Health Care" includes, for example, dental and other professional health services, durable medical equipment, etc. "Other Health Spending" includes, for example, administration and net cost of private health insurance, public health activity, research, structures and equipment, etc.

Source: Kaiser Family Foundation using data from Centers for Medicare and Medicaid Services

According to this chart, 87% of the care in the United States is spent on reactive care for those that are sick.

At the end of all of these statistics, with the sobering emphasis on more dollars spent, more insurance costs incurred, and an economy that must compete globally, the employer/plan sponsor must stop and consider: What are we getting for all of the money we are spending?

At the same time that these questions are being asked, more people are losing their jobs and their employer-based health coverage. These people forfeit chronic care for acute symptomatic care, resulting in higher rates of conditions related to their chronic illness and more emergency treatments, behavioral health impact, and poorer outcomes, in general. Communities, overall, get sick.

Couple this statistic with the economics of the global market, the recent downturn for American businesses, and our country actively evaluating the United States healthcare system as a whole. What one sees is a renewed emphasis on the intersection of healthcare costs and financial security for all of the stakeholders, as well as an evaluation of the value of each dollar spent in healthcare.

The real questions that every employer and plan sponsor, every health plan and benefits manager, should be asking must reframe the question: How much health, instead of healthcare, are we buying? How much could we buy with the same money we are spending now if we purchased services more wisely?

Understanding that things had to change if employers were to be able to continue to afford healthcare, a few forward-thinking payers and influencers began to rethink their healthcare strategies. Two healthcare "experiments" began to take hold: One involved refocusing their employees on the virtues of health and wellness and the other focused on decreasing the financial barrier to some of the care that would actually put healthier people back to work because they were compliant with their treatments.

These natural experiments that utilized reductions in co-pays for some populations continued to broaden with the inclusion of incentives for participation in annual or baseline health risk assessments, health fairs and disease management. So began the development of behavior change through incentives that actively engage consumers to participate in their health and healthcare. Today, there are hundreds of such "experiments" going on throughout the employer and health plan world. The use of these incentives, and later, disincentives—all of which have grown into the levers population health change—drives a series of questions on evidence and efficacy:

- Do they work?

- What works best?

- Under what conditions do they work?

- How do I start and how do I keep up the momentum?

This book will help you to answer some of the questions that will take you to the new culture of health. Please remember there is no one simple answer, as any or all of the levers should ONLY be used when the data shows the priority and opportunity for improvement. What we are hoping is that you will take this information and create a roadmap that makes the best sense for your organization. We welcome you to join us on this journey that we call *Leveraging Health.*

"We have a history of restricting access while hoping for better outcomes. In most cases, this has not worked to our advantage. While controlling health care expenditures seems to be the primary focus of most health care reform discussions, cost containment efforts must not produce preventable decreases in the quality of care delivered. The implementation of "fiscally responsible, clinically sensitive" Value-Based Designs restores attention to health in the health care reform debate and will ultimately produce enhanced health outcomes for the money spent. It's much more than any kind of "free" treatment—to survive, we must produce relevant benefit designs that focus on collaborative engagement for total economic and health improvement. Anything less will be ineffective."

A. MARK FENDRICK, MD
PROFESSOR, INTERNAL MEDICINE AND HEALTH
MANAGEMENT & POLICY
CO-DIRECTOR,
CENTER FOR VALUE-BASED INSURANCE DESIGN
UNIVERSITY OF MICHIGAN

Chapter 2

BEGINNING TO ASK
NEW QUESTIONS

"If we are to find the true value in value-based designs, we must extend our business-case evaluation beyond healthcare costs, and include impacts on absence, presenteeism and health-related productivity."

THOMAS PARRY, PH.D.
PRESIDENT
INTEGRATED BENEFITS INSTITUTE

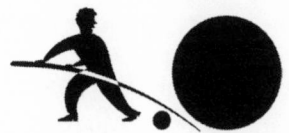

The shock factor that occurs when one considers the history of health cost inflation causes a momentary pause, at least. The connection of health to every aspect of wealth emerges, and suddenly there are new questions to ask:

What could those healthcare dollars buy that would benefit my company, my community, my family?

- How can I drive more value for every dollar that I/we spend on health?

- How can I purchase units of health instead of healthcare? After all, when I buy a car, I don't purchase units of car care, I purchase units of car work (it transports me to my job, my home, my errands, my school)—it does its job. When I hire people to work for my company, I expect them to work—not to consume healthcare.

- Have I been asking the right questions, purchasing the right products? Have I worked collaboratively with my service providers (health plan, benefits consultants, disability managers, EAP vendors, others) to ensure the health of my workforce, instead of the healthcare?

When the shock wears off, and the reality of healthcare costs v. health improvement sets in, the renegades step forward. These are the people who see a better way to create health within their workforce and their community. They consider basic behavior change strategies that can move people and groups of people to change their behaviors from unhealthy to healthy. And they look behind the closed doors, into the black boxes, and around every corner for the expansion of health in their workforce, instead of the expansion of healthcare. These renegades begin to innovate.

2.1   Innovation Drives New Direction

Once the new questions begin to form, new solutions rise to the surface. If the employer does not have the information on the general population to make health a priority, he or she must seek it. If the employer does not know where the direct medical claims are consumed (through hospital days? Emergency department visits? disability days or safety-workers' compensation costs?), then the answer must be sought.

Accepting the advice of key advisors, without integrating the total picture of health and productivity for the organization, is like driving the car without the rear axle. It won't go far and the costs to repair will be quite high.

So the renegade begins to question using different language and insisting on benchmarks for future success. Some of the questions include:

- How do I compare my total health spend with others? Can the ratio of total health dollars to the total revenue of the corporation get key leadership to embrace the change needed? If we can reduce the ratio AND improve the outcome, how do I evaluate the current benefits against the "future" benefits?

- How do I sharpen my financial acuity so that I see dividends for every health dollar that I spend?

- How will connecting that acuity and laser-focus improve the overall health of my organization so that we can compete in the markets we serve?

- How will I gain that expertise, that acuity? What outcomes need to change? How do I shift from "hold down cost" to "improve outcomes and productivity?"

- How will I get my workers to shift their behavior to deliver better health management and increase productivity while reducing health absences?

- Who has the answers I need to make these decisions? Does my health plan share appropriate information with the pharmacy manager? With the behavioral health team? With the safety and risk department and the benefits team? Who else has the information that I can use? And who is sharing this with the physicians and clinicians and holding them accountable for improved health?

- How long will it take to achieve modest improvements in financial trend? When can I see larger improvements and what will it take to get there?

These questions often divide the decision-makers into two camps: The enraged (what were we paying for?) and the engaged (how can we do better?). The engaged become the renegades, the innovators. They seek value for their health investments. This is the segment that generates the success stories in value-based designs, using levers to change the outcomes.

Two key messages keep emerging in the renegade population:

- Within our benefit portfolios, cost-shifts actually reduce total wealth, creating conservation mode. If we keep shifting costs to our employees and their families, they will not deliver any different outcome than they have over the past 20 years—they will continue to use health-care. We want them to improve their health and deliver health units—productivity—to our company.

- Outcomes happen in hopeful, controllable, competent arenas. People have to believe they can achieve better health, see the path to achieve it (including the access and affordability), and make changes to achieve it. Making behavior changes should not be so hard that most people give up, because this actually costs us money.

> "The bottom line for improving health and productivity in the workplace is about aligned incentives for the total value of health. It's no accident it's called the bottom line. Putting the person into the Culture of Health drives better outcomes for everyone."
>
> *Gregg Kamas*
> *Director of Health Risk Management*
> *IMA of Colorado, Inc.*

Renegades want change for the better. Doing the same thing over and over again—creating barriers to good health management—will not deliver good health management. It delivers poor health management, frustration, and lower productivity. Renegades change the lexicon and renegades get a different suite of solutions. Renegades become the front-line of engaged change agents. They drive innovation. They create *Cultures of Health*.

2.2 New questions drive a new suite of solutions

Once engaged, the Change Agent Renegade begins to develop a suite of solutions to answer his or her questions.

- Who has the data that will show me the total cost of healthcare at my worksite?

  Culling data from the health plan, health system, county-level reporting, service vendors (disability, workers' comp, safety-risk management, EAP) to map the trends becomes extremely important to the onset of discovery. The Renegade seeks information from every health service provider and across every business silo possible.

- What does the data show me?

  The Renegade now seeks new ways of looking at the data. Comparing trends year-over-year for increases in the general population, in segments of the populations (male v. female, under 30 years of age and over 30/over 50/etc, zip codes/counties, salary, even physician group/hospital provider) can all yield information that is worthy of consideration.

- What behaviors need to change to improve the trend line? We must flatten the curve to create better financial health.

The Renegade has just emerged from the thinking arena and has transformed into the Innovator. The solutions used before aren't working, so new solutions must be tried. Using basic tenets of behavior change, the Innovator considers the barriers to the behaviors needed and how incentives can work to break the barriers.

The Renegade is motivated by one more key question: <u>**How much excess productivity do we have and how much can we afford to lose in the marketplace?**</u> Of course, the answer to this one is, ZERO. The Renegade knows that the company is leaking productivity, and that leak has to be fixed for better performance.

Chapter 3

DIFFERENTIATING HEALTH BENEFITS FROM HEALTH INCENTIVES

"It was a simple idea: We reviewed the care patterns for gaps and opportunities. I asked the doctors what they would do if they were in my shoes. We asked employees what they knew about their health. Then, using what they said, we implemented an incentive-driven plan that engaged our doctors and patients (our members) in more rational continuing care. They saw their physicians, asked more questions, took more of their medications, told their coaches about their successes, and began to purchase health services more wisely. Suddenly, we saw our health indicators going up and our health cost trends going down. We saved money the very first year and it's continued now for three years."

JERRY REEVES, MD
CHIEF MEDICAL OFFICER
H.E.R.E.I.U. WELFARE FUNDS

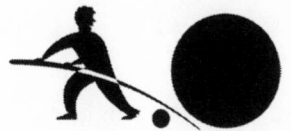

Before exploring the recent changes and experiments in benefit design, it is important to differentiate between a benefit and an incentive:

A benefit is, in effect, a contract between the plan sponsor and the individual. It spells out the *who, what* and *how much* of the agreement between the plan sponsor and the person who seeks to have medical coverage in the plan. The terms of this agreement are in effect for the entire coverage period and, generally speaking, may not be unilaterally changed by the plan sponsor during this coverage term.

An incentive is a different way the plan sponsor can change behavior. It may be initiated, or terminated at any time during a period of coverage and is generally administered outside of the standard claims payment process. As we will see in our examples, incentives, combined with an effective value-based design, are powerful tools in achieving population health improvement.

Two major factors impact the overall cost of a medical benefit plan: The scope of covered medical conditions and services, and the extent to which the plan participants use these services. This latter factor is clearly influenced not only by the medical status of the participants, but also by their care management and care-seeking behavior. It is exactly this behavior that is relevant to the discussion of value-based benefits.

Cost-sharing is an integral part of healthcare benefit design and is, in most cases, the single most powerful tool used by benefit managers to control costs. Employers can influence the amount and type of coverage purchased by an employee by having employees share in the annual cost, or premium, for coverage. By displaying *price tags,* the employer has an opportunity to communicate the value of the benefit and, at the same time, encourage enrollment in cost-effective plans. Practical experience has shown that as the employee-paid portion of coverage rises, employees either dis-enroll in high-cost plans or opt-out of their employer's coverage altogether.

Plan designers use deductibles, co-insurance and co-pays to influence utilization and costs within the medical plan. Co-payments are limited to a fixed dollar amount and, in general, may have an effect on utilization. In contrast, co-insurance, since it reflects a percentage of the acquisition cost of the service or product, may amount to a significant sum, and is definitely a deterrent to utilization of high-cost medications and services.

Deductibles, if high enough, will totally deter utilization. By having the participant have some skin in the game, designers are expecting that the individual will become a better consumer of healthcare and steer their utilization towards services and products that are effective.

Moreover, by minimizing their cost-sharing expense, it is assumed individuals will make decisions that will lower overall expense for the plan sponsor. Underlying all of these tools is the assumption that the individual will pro-actively seek effective medical care and, as a result of the plan design, will choose the most cost-efficient means of managing their health. The reality may be quite different.

3.1 The Rand Health Insurance Experiment

In the early 1970s, the RAND Institute undertook an 11-year population-based study to help understand the impact of varying levels of cost-sharing on health plan cost and health-seeking behavior. Large numbers of participants were randomly assigned to medical plans with levels of co-insurance varying from free to 95%. Participants' health status was evaluated annually during the term of their enrollment (generally from four-five years). Not surprisingly, the researchers clearly demonstrated that higher levels of cost-sharing led to decreased use of the healthcare system. Elimination of cost-sharing encouraged more medical care but, interestingly, the researchers were unable to demonstrate that this increase in medical care led to better health outcomes.[4]

Some benefit designers have seized on these findings to advance the idea that health plans should incorporate significant levels of cost-sharing. In effect, these new designers recast the results to say that shifting costs to the participant is beneficial to the plan sponsor and that it does not have adverse effects for those enrolled in the plan.

Before accepting this idea, it's perhaps wise to take a more thorough look at the results of the RAND study. First, the study must be placed in context. During the study time period, the role of chronic disease and condition management was little understood. In fact, apart from some medications used to treat hypertension and heart failure, little or no pharmaceuticals were available to help control chronic conditions. Further, physicians and other caregivers did not extensively practice preventive medicine. This is a stark difference from today's healthcare environment where we recognize the ongoing impact of chronic medical conditions and have deployed an array of interventions to address primary prevention as well as ongoing management of chronic disease.

Co-insurance was also the only cost-sharing methodology used in the experiment. Moreover, this occurred during a period we spoke about earlier, where cost-sharing only applied to medical/surgical treatments and out-of-pocket maximums were in place to protect participants from catastrophic costs. Pharmaceuticals were totally the responsibility of the patient with no cost-sharing. Subsequent research, conducted by Dana Goldman at RAND, showed that doubling co-pays for chronic disease medications leads first to significant reductions in use of these medications (consistent with the original study) and then to marked increases in medical costs due to increased use of emergency room and hospital admissions.[5]

Despite the large numbers of participants, the researchers acknowledge that the study design did not allow for sufficient sample size, or follow-up duration, to produce valid results for certain populations, including children, low-income groups, and those with cancer or chronic medical conditions. The most problematic finding involves the decreasing utilization. Both effective and non-effective services were curtailed as co-insurance rose. There is no evidence that faced with economic consequences, participants shifted their utilization to those services that enhanced health and decreased use of non-effective care. It is this last find-ing that led one author, R.H. Brook, writing in the *Journal of the American Medical Association* to postulate that the role of benefits ought to be restructured to facilitate access to highly effective treatments.[6] In effect, this article is the fore-runner to today's *Value-Based Benefit Design.*

It is with this knowledge and the challenges that employers and health plans are facing in today's environment that we share with you the insurance and health experiments that are evolving today along the *Health Value Continuum*, where innovators share results and challenges in their efforts to purchase units of health and improve productivity of the workforce and communities.

Chapter 4

LEVERS ARE THE PERFORMANCE TUNERS

"The City of Springfield, Oregon has a Wellness Mission: We are in partnership to pursue a healthy, productive and balanced lifestyle through a variety of wellness opportunities in a fun, encouraging, and safe atmosphere. Most of us do not get refreshing sleep; we eat too much, work too hard, and find too little time for fun, friends and family.

The City's health risk appraisal information shows depression as a major expense to the City. That elevated depression is a focus for value-based levers. A value challenge to the City is to encourage health in the area of depression, as well as in an overall balanced lifestyle. We showed we could reduce total costs through a value-based design for diabetes. We learned we have to manage depression, so we've inserted the mission into our Culture of Health."

ARDIS BELKNAP
HUMAN RESOURCES MANAGER
CITY OF SPRINGFIELD, OR

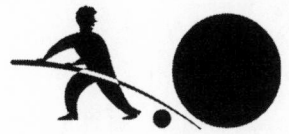

Levers have been used for thousands of years to move a large object from its current station. The importance of a lever in population health is that it can move a group of people into a new health status without hands-on contact, thus preserving privacy and encouraging self-management of one's health.

As we addressed in previous chapters, the issue in the marketplace in the early 21st century was one of escalating costs in health management. Health costs had been rising and managed care had not been able to sustainably contain the costs of over-consumption and rising chronic disease.

In the employer community, there was no doubt that health costs had to be controlled as they were escalating beyond the GDP and beyond employer profitability. Shareholder value was decreasing as more companies experienced double-digit health cost inflation with single-digit profitability. In simple terms, the force of healthcare cost inflation, if not modified, was going to threaten the competitive ability of American enterprises. The actions taken to date had not sustainably reduced the health cost trends.

4.1 The Emergence of Innovation: Levers

Innovators use data to develop an integrated suite of plan design features and incentives that will incrementally improve the health management of populations. In the employer arena, privacy becomes a key concept in managing health. The employer looks at populations, not people, and tracks the inappropriate healthcare use and trend lines. Then, design changes are implemented in benefits and in incentives. These are the LEVERS.

What is a Lever?

A lever is a device that transmits or modifies force or motion.

In its classic form, a lever is a rigid bar that pivots about one point and is used to move an object at a second point by force applied at a third. It is one of six simple machines (lever, pulley, wheel and axle, pulley screw, wedge and incline plane) that form the basis for more complex machines, moving production lines and improving development of new products and services.

Levers can also be defined as a means of persuading or achieving an end, such as leveraging a plan to improve productivity.

Levers can be considered the *fine tuners* for better performance. If the employer does not have all the data on the health status of the population, then a health risk appraisal (HRA) can be used to fill in the gaps—and an incentive can be put into place to coax the completion of the HRA. If a segment of the population is using the emergency department for asthma treatment instead of staying true to their inhaler regimen, perhaps a co-pay reduction for medication could work to get many of the folks back into appropriate treatment. If there are too many MRIs being used, particularly without evidence in the recognized medical literature that the MRI is even needed for treatment, then a raise in the co-pay—a disincentive—can be put into place to defer some of the use.

Think of the levers as the tuners that drive a better use of gasoline in the engine. Car idling poorly? Tune it. Car jerks when the gas pedal is depressed? Tune it. Each of these "tuners" adjusts the behavior of the car. That's a lever: A tuner for better performance, like the magic of music when all the parts work harmoniously to achieve the better outcome. Stereo tuners, iPod tuners, car tuners, population tuners—levers to drive efficiency, reduce errors, improve outcomes, and make the instrument sing. Levers can be used to reduce the overall financial investment in the running of the car or the sound of the violin, or the health of the population. [7]

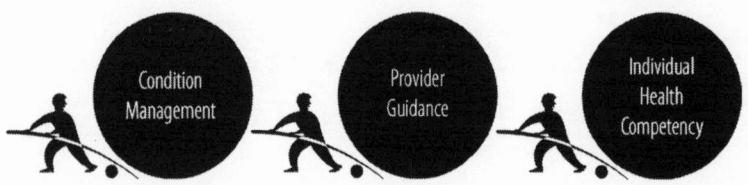

INNOVATOR KEVIN O'Brien, CEO of Partners in Care, a physician organization in New Jersey.

"According to Wikipedia, **Performance tuning** is the improvement of _system_ _performance_. This is typically a computer application, but the same methods can be applied to economic markets, bureaucracies or other complex systems."

At Partners in Care, we began to witness parallels between computer network performance tuning, organizational performance tuning, and health benefit management performance tuning as early as 2004.

Essentially, performance tuning involves identifying key metrics tied to a complex process or system, studying the interrelationships of these key metrics, identifying the balance or harmony points, and adjusting strategies, in essence adjusting key levers, to optimize the performance of the system.

In the case of healthcare, these items are sourced to individual populations, the actual participants in the delivery system, the health benefit administrators, and the corporate benefit managers. Because the combinations of the variables within these four macro-categories are virtually infinite, no two populations can be addressed in exactly the same way. We have found that robust use of data analysis to identify the metrics for specific populations as they interface with their macro environment is key to identifying the proper levers and lever positions for optimizing the performance (read: health behaviors) of the specific population.

> *For example, a Diabetes Disease Management program will do little to assist an organization whose population has less than 1% of their people diagnosed with diabetes but spends 70% of its healthcare dollars on pregnancy-related expenditures.*
>
> *Conversely, maternity benefits will do little for a medium-sized professional firm whose average age is 55 and has little to no exposure to pregnancy related initiatives; nor will the latter firm be sensitized to the medical malpractice issues compressing availability of obstetricians.*
>
> *The key to success is to use the data to identify and optimize the three to five key initiatives which will be core to the environment in question, and then to implement the initiatives with a rigorous, dispassionate, metric-driven feedback loop to ensure the initiatives can evolve and adapt.*

4.2   EUREKA! Finding the value in health

Building on our cumulative expertise (we, the authors, are two physicians and a gerontologist), there was a collective understanding that some companies were achieving success in modifying health risks within their organizations. Innovators tend to share experiences and challenges, and innovators in businesses were no exception. To this end, a survey was developed, lists of companies and contacts were accumulated based upon mutual contacts, and phone surveys were begun.

A 12-question screening survey was designed that would identify the organization size, number of covered lives, annual revenues, experience in disease and condition management, sophistication in data management, culture and involvement of the leadership in health management and behavior change. This survey would build upon previous healthcare trend surveys showing the movement and evolution from the Fee for Service to the HMO market to the PPO, Consumer-Directed Health Plans, and Pay for Performance efforts. Surveys were conducted one-on-one by phone, and the responses captured in a simple database that could be graphed. The screening survey was successful in capturing data elements, but it was the story of innovation that was revealed through the surveys that proved the most beneficial; innovators were eager to share the challenges and successes in changing cultures of entitlement to cultures of worksite health improvement.[8]

The early outreach was daunting—some people were slow to share, and the first interviews were conducted with folks who had long-held relationships with the interviewer. Yet, there was a movement afloat.[9]

The interviews were designed to gain comparative information as to what benefits designs and changes were implemented to create better—and more appropriate—use of the healthcare system. What resulted was the clear delineation of companies on a three-part path to improvement: Some were just beginning, typically using reduced or waived co-pays for prevention and wellness screenings; some had moved into a value-based design space, using reduced or waived co-pays for diabetes management, mimicking early success from the experiences at Pitney Bowes and Asheville NC; some were managing co-pay reductions across several chronic diseases plus onsite services, total data integration, environmental change (healthy foods in vending machines, behavioral change support, etc.) and company leadership support. The graph of the Health Value Continuum shows the movement in its earliest stages in 2007.

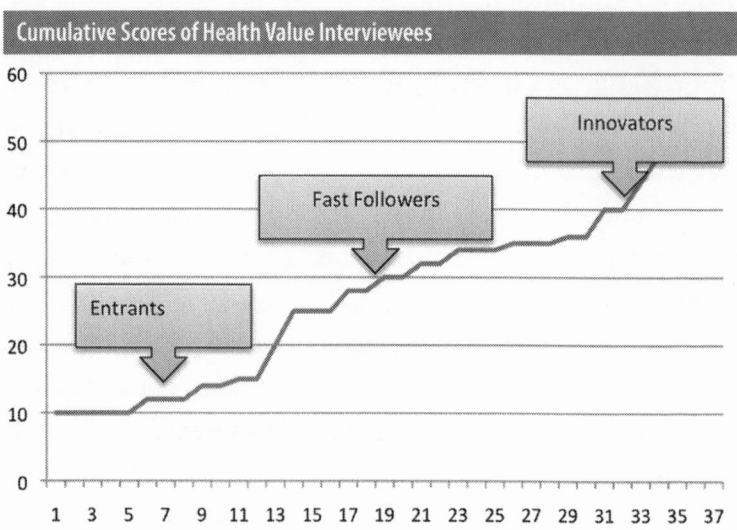

Phone interviews with 36 companies through 2007 were scored on a scale from 0 to 50.

4.3 What the Surveys Told Us

Through these interviews we found a number of both broad and very specific findings. In the broadest terms, the number of companies initializing the utilization of these levers has increased dramatically over the three years. Most of the early adopter companies interviewed were large self-funded employers. Over time, the types of organizations/companies utilizing these levers have expanded. There are more government entities (cities/counties/ states) as employers tested the value-based concepts with success, and there are smaller companies—as small as 100 employees— moving into the space. Along with the expansion of companies utilizing value- based design, there are also new products and services to assist the adoption of value-based designs [the Center for Health Value Innovation has named the technologies V-BIT for value-based information technologies].

The survey also found that the interviewed companies showed a variety of innovations and implementation strategies. These activities are often integrated into the health management activities of each company.

Many of the organizations are able to review their data on medical claims, pharmacy and lab costs, disability days, and behavioral health costs, even if they cannot integrate all the data at the patient level.

To date, 104 levers have been catalogued by the Center for Health Value Innovation [hereinafter known as the Center]. Some of these were similar in that the action was the same but the conditions that they were being focused on were different i.e., labs/exams for diabetes and labs/exams for asthma. The early use of levers was focused on care and costs associated with chronic conditions. The levers were utilized to change consumer/

patient purchasing and persistence to prescribed medications for chronic conditions. The reasoning was a gap in care that was driving costs for the organizations. The levers then expanded, or "shifted to the left," to include more prevention and wellness interventions. Some of these levers were tied to out-of-pocket costs for medications, premium costs, or health savings accounts. A final suite of levers emerged to direct consumers and patients to cost and efficiency-sensitive providers—such as onsite services, convenience case clinics, even medical travel—and often provide incentives to the service providers (physicians, nurse practitioners, hospital systems) for providing the time and effort to engage the consumer/patient.

The initial discovery of the levers also revealed that they were disorganized in their use. Most companies began the use of the levers, or plan designs and incentives, based upon academic evidence or anecdotal information from other employers, and then bravely broadened the efforts. In some instances, there was little focus as to the suitability of the intervention for the particular company's experience—many tried the "diabetes management" approach without quantifying the potential investment or the actual incidence of the disease in their population.

Current Risk/Waste Reduction
- Delete unnecessary use
- Improve chronic care treatment and persistence

Future Risk Reduction
- Identify and manage emerging risk
- Compress illness and push it into the future

Individual Health Competency
- Lifestyle change
- Goal setting and reporting

The disorganization has evolved into a very organized system of priorities. At the core is a focus on current risk management or waste reduction. In this entry, present risks that can be positively modified are identified and interventions are quantified to lead to priorities for implementation. If a person never fills the first prescription, or is scheduled for a blood draw and never gets it, or fills three but not all 12 of the prescriptions for a year's worth of care, then there is waste. This is current risk, just as surely as not having any clinical exams is current risk, just as surely as not getting the flu shot if one has heart disease is also current risk. These first levers do still usually focus on chronic disease management, particularly diabetes, as most of the seminars and editorials have focused on this disease—it has a well accepted set of national guidelines for quality care, and a finite set of measures and metrics to show success, such as cholesterol and hypertension screening and goals along with HbA1C, foot and kidney screenings. Appropriate care in these measures has shown a reduction in both direct and indirect health costs.

The second tier of intervention focuses on the future, emerging risks—the risks that prevention and wellness exams can help to identify. By reducing the emerging risk, that which is not known because a person did not receive a wellness exam or biometric screen that links to a condition, the aggregate information of total health risk to the organization can be quantified and education, screenings, and incentives can be put into place that help consumers better manage their own health. In smaller companies, particularly those that are fully-insured, this often acts as an entry point in the value-based design arena, with their concentration of efforts in chronic conditions at a later date. Either entry point does work. Corporate culture, company-specific data and company business goals should be utilized in order to decide on the best area for initial attention.

The third tier for plan sponsors is that of employee/consumer engagement for individual health improvement, the ultimate in value-based design. In this tier, communications that are consumer-driven and focused are used to improve patient account ability as well as organizational accountability. The consumer identifies his/her health improvement goals and these goals are linked to those of the employer/plan sponsor. They are reinforced with messaging, design and incentives that can be subtle as well as direct, and these can range from healthier choices in the cafeteria to Personal Health Record use, to stress management—but they all circle back to the goals that are consumer-defined. This makes Lever Group 3—Individual Health Competency, the consumer-driven plan at its best.

4.4 Replicability and Scalability

In 2008, the authors began asking for business-based evidence and outcomes from the companies who had responded to the initial survey and subsequent dialogues. This evidence is built upon benefit consultant input to these companies, some actuarial models, and, in a few cases, academic review of the experiences—and then they are downloaded into the Center's database. These metrics have been aligned with some of the levers, and new efforts are beginning to quantify the effect of single levers and/or suites of levers to change population behaviors. At the end of the day, the goal of getting people to acknowledge their responsibility in their own health management, make more informed decisions on cost and effectiveness of treatment, and follow their physician's orders for managing their health has shown results in decreased emergency room visits, decrease in unplanned absenteeism, improved screening processes and improved health status [defined as reduction in risk levels, reduction in co-morbid complications related to under-managed conditions, improved productivity measures, improved function across many conditions, and early successful intervention for cancers, heart disease, and so forth). This is the true promise of the levers of value-based design: Improved health and quality of life for people and communities plus reduced total finances inappropriately spent on healthcare instead of health improvement.

There is now a clearly defined set of levers that influence behaviors across the spectrum of keeping the healthy behaviors intact, lowering the number of risks, managing the acute and chronic care, and creating sustainable clinical and financial health. The 104 levers have been rolled up into 15 macro levers. In the chapters to follow we will showcase how the 15 levers are used and encourage the development of more innovation in the kinds of levers, the suites of levers, and the measures of dividends.

UNDERSTANDING THE LEVERS

"I like to say, 'It ain't dog food if the dog don't eat it'. Of course, when it comes to changing our personal health behavior, not all dogs like the same food. The key is finding the right food for the right dog when and where they are hungry. The big secret is that we have the tools to do exactly that."

NEAL SOFIAN
DIRECTOR BEHAVIORAL INTERVENTIONS
RESOLUTION HEALTH

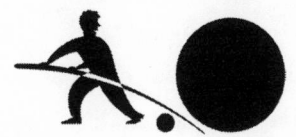

In chapter four, the concept of a lever was discussed and the organization of the discovery was laid out. It's now time to understand the deeper significance and the drivers of the levers—what drove the implementation, where are they used, and how do they work?

5.1 The Rise of Value-Based Design

The emergence of value-based designs, particularly in the benefit design for improved health management, was driven through the iconic experiences at Pitney Bowes and Asheville NC (for more information, visit *www.vbhealth.org*). The concept that was utilized by both these employers, as well as some of the other early innovators, included a four-step process that included collecting and utilizing data to identify opportunities for improvement within the organization. The data looked for vulnerable populations, populations whose status could be improved through some behavior change; applied levers—benefit plan design and incentives—to move the most vulnerable populations; measured the improvement of behavior change and emerging opportunities to improve the management and outcomes; and quantified the dividend (improved quality, health and reduction in financial trend) to the individual and the company.

The following diagram showcases the four-step process[10]:

Value-based design is a tool that is part of an evidence-based approach to managing health outcomes.

- Uses data *to*

- Invest in benefit designs and programs *that*

- Change behaviors through appropriate resources *to*

- Improve Quality, Health, Productivity and Financial Outcomes (Dividend)

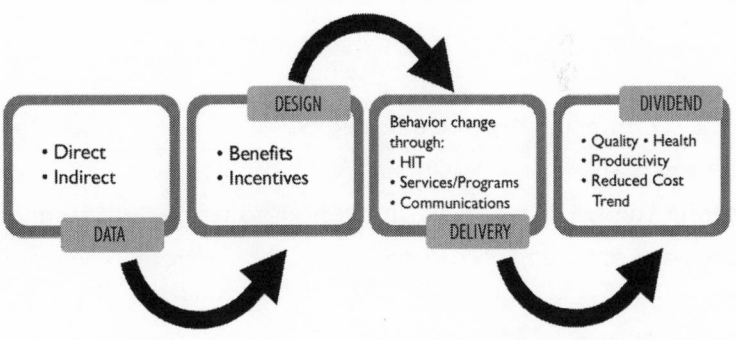

(c) 2009 Center for Health Value Innovation

The value-based design movement escalated as a result of the efforts of a group of innovators from several arenas:

- Experts from Pitney Bowes and Asheville NC

- Academic information from Mark Fendrick, MD and Michael Chernew, PhD, co-founders of the Center for Value-Based Insurance Design at the University of Michigan

- Academic and peer-reviewed information from Rand Institute, Health Affairs, and other noteworthy journals

- National thought leaders from health plans/pharmacy benefit management companies, consumer engagement experts, hospital systems and provider organizations; and the focused outreach from the Center for Health Value Innovation, a non-profit established to identify the innovators in the market and create an information exchange that would fuel new innovation in value.

5.2   The Full Impact of Levers

Levers can build confidence in the health management team of the employer, the service providers and the workforce. The levers are defined within the four-step value-based process of DATA, DESIGN, DELIVERY, DIVIDENDS (see diagram above):

- DATA: Can the data be sequenced and predictive/benchmarked at the business-relevant level? What can we achieve in one year, in three years?

- DESIGN: Should the levers be:

  - preventive (keep risk from forming, or reduce the rate at which health costs cause financial risk to the organization?)

° sequenced (first we insist on an HRA, then a biometric screen, then preventive care...)

° segmented (we'll provide a co-pay reduction for preventive services such as flu shots, but only for our at-risk population, for example)

° titrated (we provide the flu shots for those with diabetes and asthma this year, then add more populations as we begin to see the financial trend reduced), and/or

° clinician inclusive (we have to include the clinician in the sharing of rewards, particularly if we're asking for more service per member)?

- DELIVERY: How do we best implement these levers? In what setting are they most likely to have the greatest impact? What outcomes are we willing to risk? To reward? How much more would it take to change the food in the vending machines? Create rewards for bi-weekly achievement of goals?

- DIVIDEND: These answers will prioritize investment and focus your efforts on expected, measurable dividends to your organization and your community

°   outcomes that will define partners/providers/partici-
    pants, and

°   outcomes that define acceptable levels of investment
    risk—VALUE

This will lead to the levers you will use in your environment, because even Innovators know that the financial pot is not un-limited—companies must start with what they can afford, learn about the impact, measure the financial trend reduction, then use the dividend of the financial trend reduction to deploy more incentives to change more behaviors. The goal is to create afford-able, accessible healthcare, using levers to modify use, disuse, and un-use—and ultimately to save jobs and compete globally.

Levers are a valuable tool for driving the population to health improvement, the community to quality outcomes, and econom-ics of health to a reduction in inflation.

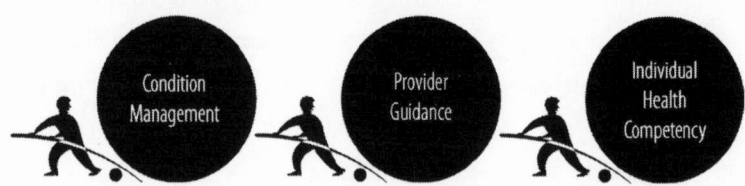

BRINGING HEALTH IMPROVEMENT INSIDE

FROM INNOVATOR FRED *Williams, Director, Health Management Strategies, Quest Diagnostics, and member of the Board of Directors of the Center for Health Value Innovation.*

Fred Williams knows the price of poor health, and, more importantly, the price of undiagnosed risk. "The business of Quest Diagnostics is to help improve the health of patients through unsurpassed diagnostic insights and innovations. The importance of our mission touched me personally a few years ago when my childhood friend, Joey, died suddenly of a heart attack on the golf course. I'm reminded of our mission much more positively when I hear from the people whose lives are touched by our wellness programs. Nearly every day, someone shares with us how the knowledge they've gained through participation in our health risk assessment - or the encouragement and information they've received through our worksite support programs - have helped improve their health or lengthen their lives. And that is quite gratifying."

As director of health management strategies, Fred's work today, along with the many wellness professionals and volunteers at Quest Diagnostics, is focused on improving employee engagement in personal health management, a key element in value-based designs. The steps to improving employee engagement and reducing personal health risk at Quest Diagnostics are designed to deliver a return on investment in the overall health of the employee population. Originally, the company had a meager response to its health risk assessment offering, with 11,000 of its 42,000 employees taking part, but only one year after Quest Diagnostics began to incent participation and actively market health improvement, that number grew to 29,000. "A key success factor," Williams explained, "was that we shifted our definition of the term 'health plan' away from plan coverage and toward personal health engagement. We wanted to help employees think beyond asking 'What am I covered for when I am sick?', and rather ask themselves 'What can I be doing to stay well?'"

Today, Quest Diagnostics has company-wide health improvement goals, which are reported on quarterly. Its program includes:

- Health promotion teams have been established at all locations. Teams are comprised of volunteers, all of whom carry a passion for their particular subject area, such as fitness, weight management, risk assessment participation, or tobacco cessation.

- Annually, employees and spouses or partners are encouraged to participate in Blueprint for Wellness™ by completing a health risk questionnaire and providing a blood sample either at an onsite wellness event, or at one of Quest Diagnostics' over 2,000 patient service centers.

- *The participants each receive a comprehensive report that integrates their health risk profile, based on their responses to health lifestyle questions, and their clinical laboratory values. The report includes current and prior lab values, lifestyle risks, and steps that can be taken to reduce those risks.*

- *The program helps to detect health risk earlier, and as a result, helps drive lower health costs. It is free to participants, and those participants who are also enrolled in the company's health plans receive a bi-weekly reduction in their insurance premium.*

Quest Diagnostics' value-based design:

- *Early adopter of a consumer-driven health plan*

- *Incentives for health risk questionnaire, biometric measurements, and clinical screenings*

- *Evidence-based guidelines for risk/disease modification*

- *Waive co-pays/co-insurance for screenings*

- *Periodic posting of employee stories of improved health, and internal wellness ambassadors support the behavior changes*

Quest Diagnostics Charts New Waters in the Culture of Health

In 2007, Quest Diagnostics took worksite prevention and wellness a step further. The company added to its employee health program an opportunity for colon cancer screening using the Insure® FIT™ test, one of the methods for colorectal cancer screening included in American Cancer Society guidelines. This test can be done without time away from work, and without dietary or medication changes. The company mailed specimen collection kits to the homes of employees over age 50 (and to African Americans over age 45), performed the laboratory testing on the specimens, and sent a results report to each participant. Any participant with a positive result received a phone call from a physician, who reviewed the results with the participant, and encouraged them to take appropriate follow up action. About 2,800 employees participated in the program's first year, and after program enhancements, participation doubled in 2008. According to medical experts, detection of colon cancer in its early stages is a key factor in survival.

Quest Diagnostics is creating a culture of health and engagement. As Williams says, "We wanted to walk the walk, so we could demonstrate that early identification and education can improve health status. It is clearly a journey, with some twists and turns, but we know that we are having a measurable effect."

Who Is Quest Diagnostics?

- *43,000 employees*

- *66,000 covered lives*

- *Annual Revenues $7.2 billion revenues reported in 2008*

- *Winner National Business Group on Health's Best Employers for Healthy Lifestyles Award for five consecutive years, most recently in 2009 with NBGH's highest level of recognition, the Platinum award.*

Chapter 6

LEVERS DRIVE PERFORMANCE IMPROVEMENT IN BEHAVIOR CHANGE

"Being able to help someone with a medical challenge is gratifying…. Being able to prevent that medical challenge is profound and core to our business…Being able to touch the lives of many is our passion…The result is a healthier, more satisfied and productive workforce resulting in the lowest possible cost."

DAVE JOHNSON MD, MBA, CPE
PRESIDENT, VIVACITY

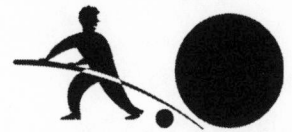

The levers drive a series of changes in the health management of the population. Each lever has a purpose (to change a behavior in a defined group of people) and performance improvement metric that is proposed at the outset (what do we think this will do?). When considering a lever or suite of levers, the benefits designer asks:

- How large is the targeted population?

- How many people will be affected positively?

- What is the risk of negative response, or unintended consequence; what is the cost and how many people would be affected?

- What is the timeframe to achieve the performance improvement?

- How will we know when we get the improvement—what is the measure (for instance, in diabetes management, reducing the co-pay for a prescription medication should lead to improved adherence, so increased numbers of refills and, potentially, improved glucose levels could be the desired metrics).

> ### What is an Incentive?
>
> An incentive is a disincentive with a marketing wrapper. Providing a reward for completing the HRA is similar to saying, "no reward without the completion." The concept in value-based design is to frame the incentive or disincentive – the lever – that will coax the population into the behavior desired.

The goals of the lever(s) should align with the overall goals of health improvement AND financial responsibility for the organization and its health plan members.

Levers can be used singly or in combinations called "suites." Each suite may affect one or more behaviors and outcomes. Levers can be part of the health benefit plan (usually installed one time per year) or can be installed as a stand-alone incentive/disincentive to fine-tune behaviors throughout the benefit year. As we said earlier, most companies do not change the benefit design during the year, but many do install incremental incentives throughout the year as the review their data and look for opportunities to "tune" the performance.

It's important to remember as you read through this chapter that levers can be positive (we will reduce your co-pay for your annual physical if you go to these physicians) or disincentives (if you go to physicians outside of the ones noted, you will pay more for your co-pay). Communication is the key—people can be guided to the proper behavior, but ultimately each person has a choice to participate in how he/she behaves. If you are worried about the use of incentives and disincentives, remember this: People are used to both incentives and disincentives—it's how they learned to be careful around a stove.

6.1 A System of Levers Drives the Process and Outcomes Desired

Through the cumulative learning experience with 80 intervie-wees, plus over 150 online surveys, we know that the levers focus on three general areas for improvement: Condition management (how do we manage chronic and acute conditions?), provider guidance (creating designs and incentives that promote evidence-based diagnosis and treatment or reduce the costs of care, such as through urgent care clinics), and individual health management (competency). Each area has a purpose for improvement, and each area has three questions that are asked for metrics and timelines.

6.2 Current Risk or Condition Management

In assessing current risk, it is important to gather the ini-tial comparative trends for medical claims, Rx claims and, if possible, lab tests. These can be overall costs, or they can be segmented by gender, age, salary, and other variables that the benefits manager defines.

The typical first question is, "What conditions are in our current highest costs, what is causing them, and how can we bring them down quickly?" The employer is looking for high-cost relief, but with this caveat: The answer lies in a total health management approach. For example, in the experience from Pitney Bowes, the original question was, "Who will cost us $10,000+ in the next three to five years, and where in our population can we see current evidence of the manageable cost of care?" This drove the discovery of undermanaged chronic conditions. In the case of the smaller employers in the Detroit Chamber of Commerce, the question was, "How can we learn what the current risk is, and where is there unknown risk within that population?" This resulted in the insertion of the health risk appraisal and contracts for change with incentives.

Condition management demands a long-term approach to improved care in order to reduce the high costs of rescue treatments, reduce the level of co-occurring conditions (co-morbid conditions, such as hypertension in the diabetic population), and promote healthier lifestyle behaviors. The most-often cited chronic conditions that cause high costs are cardiovascular conditions, cancer, diabetes, depression, asthma, and musculoskeletal conditions (back injuries, arthritis, osteoporosis, etc.).

When considering the category of current risk, there may be instances of high cost, high absenteeism or disability, high safety risk...each of these has an impact on the total health expenditures. Therefore, the levers must address the root cause of what is driving the escalation in healthcare cost.

The most typical answers are:

- Access (Is the co-pay too high? Is there a transportation problem or a scheduling problem so care is avoided?)

- Avoidance (side effects from the drug, denial of the condition, dislike of the clinician or the test)

- Relevance (I don't have a problem with circulation in my feet, even if I'm diabetic; I'm not worried if I have to get more tests or drugs—my employer pays for it).

Therefore, the levers seek to change the behaviors underlying each of these questions:

Condition Management

Goal: Create persistency – "stickiness" – to care management over time

Access	• Reduce copays for diagnosis, treatment, or tests • Bring the services onsite (screenings such as mammograms, flu shots, treatment for acute conditions such as earache and sore throat in Occupational Health settings)
Avoidance	• Remove prior authorization for certain conditions so the patient is not "turned off" by side effects of the first prescription • Create a reward for the first prescription fill of a statin medication, or for completing the foot and eye exam for diabetes
Relevance	• Provide a timeline for completion of a recommended test, then create a disincentive if it's not completed (i.e. higher copay or higher cost for the next visit) • Mandatory enrollment in condition or disease management.

The suite of levers in "Condition Management" is defined by the outcome desired. The usual outcome is to lower the health cost trend caused by under-managed or under-diagnosed conditions. The incentives and disincentives, including the changes in the benefit plan, must cause the behavior change in the desired population. For condition management, this is most-often the persistent management of chronic care.

6.3 Provider Guidance

As before, there are three prominent questions that drive the suite of levers that can alter the trend to future risk:

- Access (Are there enough Primary Care Physicians (PCPs) to treat the community? If not, can nurse practitioners or onsite clinics fill the void? Additionally, will the PCPs accept new patients—and can an incentive be put into place that will cause them to accept new patients?)

- Avoidance (I don't need to go see the doctor, it's just my asthma acting up)

- Relevance (I only take advice from my doctor, and he didn't tell me to get that test)

Physicians and aligned care providers can be extremely helpful in early detection, long-term persistency to chronic care, and behavior change. Creating benefits designs and incentives that link the provider community to the improved outcomes of the employed population may be the focus of an employer's strategy to change and improve behaviors. Some of the levers in provider guidance could be:

Provider Guidance
Goal: Create meaningful, timely, actionable interaction with appropriate providers

Access	• Improve reimbursement to providers who practice with evidence-based guidelines • Reduce copays for use of urgent care clinics instead of emergency rooms, or increase out-of-pocket expenses for use of ER
Avoidance	• Create an incentive for consultation with the pharmacist, EAP counselor, or lifestyle coach.
Relevance	• Create an incentive for travel to a medical center of excellence for treatment

The use of tied incentives between the individual and the clinician is an extremely important suite of levers for improved health and financial outcomes. The tie of the patient/consumer to the doctor, pharmacist, and other professionals is one of the most trusted bonds in medicine and health management. By reducing the cost and avoidance barriers at the consumer level, and improving the reimbursement levels for more time spent with the most vulnerable folks in the physician office, for example, an aligned strategy is formed that coaxes the consumer into better health management techniques.

6.4   Individual Health/Competency

People learn basic life skills including health management throughout their life; some are more interested in these skills than others. In order to create persistent health management and reduce risk to each person and the organization, a level of personal health competency and individual responsibility is imperative. All organizations must look at what the lifestyle, prevention, and wellness behaviors of their population are in order to discern what new skills are necessary for improvement and what existing skills have been pushed aside—these may need to be renewed.

The question set for individual health/competency includes not only direct accountability for personal health improvement, but also includes the behaviors that affect financial, social, and environmental responsibility that inevitably influence health. These include managing expenses and planning for retirement (hence the use of a flexible spending account or a health savings account); attachment to a peer group (inside or outside one's employment) that provides encouragement and support (friends, family, church groups, volunteer organizations, etc.), and a respect for community. If these and other direct health behaviors are not managed well, the chronic care and the future risk will not be managed well, either.

In the three questions, the causes of neglect to personal health vary:

1. Access (Is there a primary care clinician available for my annual exam? What is the co-pay for my exam, and is it affordable? I do not have access to exercise equipment or to public parks. I do not have access to healthy foods at work.)
2. Avoidance (I do not have time for online record keeping or goal-setting, I don't have time to take care of myself, I am too busy.)
3. Relevance (I see no reason for my employer to know my health risks; I have no need for counseling for my smoking, my drinking; I don't need exercise, I still fit in my clothes)

Individual Competency

Goal: Create accountability for personal and organizational health

Access
- Reduce copay for annual physical
- Waive copay for colorectal screening

Avoidance
- Deposit more dollars into Health Savings Account for people who use their Personal Health Records to set goals and manage their fitness
- Increase insurance premiums for smokers who refuse to enroll in a cessation program

Relevance
- Charge a higher insurance premium for those who fail to complete their health risk appraisals or who fail to enroll in an appropriate condition or disease management program

Creating the teachable moment in personal health management and creating competency in long-term personal health improvement are strategies that are not new. What is new is that employers are recognizing that these are important pieces to the total health approach. They are skills that are transportable— they do leave with the individual if the individual leaves—but they also accelerate the worksite into a culture of health. The more competent, persistent, and literate the population, the more that health cost trends can be reduced.

From Innovator Michael Taylor, MD, Medical Director for Health Promotion at Caterpillar, and Chairman of the Board of the Center for Health Value Innovation, 2009.

Caterpillar's health and productivity strategy began in the mid-1990's with the implementation of exclusive hospital contracting and development of a specific Caterpillar physician network (PPO). Corporate Medical and Benefit Design experts soon recognized both the value of the network and the fact this would not be sufficient to control healthcare costs. In 1997, Caterpillar's health promotion initiative was launched with the goal of helping Caterpillar employees and their families make healthier lifestyle choices and make better healthcare decisions.

By 2002, the annual healthcare cost trend was averaging 4%. This level of inflation was not acceptable to Caterpillar leadership, so new initiatives were launched to maintain annual healthcare cost trends at less than the consumer price index. This required an increased effort in the areas of health promotion, pharmacy and plan design innovation. These efforts ultimately have resulted in an annual trend of <2% from 2002 through 2008.

One area of need was to help our population with diabetes. This has been a two-pronged effort. Using results from the

Steno Diabetes Trial, a program was implemented to control the cardiovascular risk factors among those with diabetes, thus preventing the major cause of morbidity and mortality and those afflicted with diabetes.

The second effort was to identify those at risk for developing diabetes and apply the lessons learned from the Diabetes Prevention Trials published from Finland and the United States. Over 2,500 employees, spouses and retirees with diabetes or at risk for developing diabetes have been involved in the program. We are seeing better control of cardiovascular risk factors such as blood pressure, lipids and physical activity.

We identified a simple biometric measure that is predictive of insulin resistance, a key risk factor for heart disease and diabetes. This measure is used to identify risk groups and enroll them into the program.

The intervention model is based on the concept of self-efficacy, or helping employees through education and training, to develop the confidence they need to take care of their diabetes and work with their physicians confidently. Tools are provided for the participants to decide upon goals and present them to their physician for agreement. The concept is that the physician provides the expertise and direction; our program provides the tools for the patient and physician to be successful. Our program drives participants to the physician with evidence-based recommendations, thereby involving the physician in the participants' care at the point of service.

Metrics have evolved to better reflect the goals of the program. We use a composite measure for diabetes that includes HbAIC, Blood Pressure, LDL cholesterol, Smoking status and Aspirin therapy as our primary measure of success, thus focusing on clinical outcomes rather than process measures.

Chapter 7

PERFORMANCE TUNING WITH LEVERS DELIVERS RESULTS

"To create an environment where employees are both motivated and empowered to fully engage and take action requires creative and insightful messaging, supported by examples of proven success. In these environments, those who have had success in improving their own health have the opportunity to champion local programs, and even mentor individuals in need of support, and, in turn, help to create more success stories."

BILL GERMANAKOS
WINNER, NBC SEASON 4 "THE BIGGEST LOSER"
DIRECTOR, CORPORATE WELLNESS, QUEST DIAGNOSTICS INC.

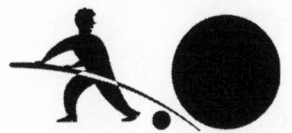

Once the data is accumulated and the priorities for intervention are set, the range of levers must be considered. Controlling for current risk is the first place to start. Remember, not all dividends occur in the short term—the outcome desired, and the effort needed for sustainable change, will drive the time needed for dividends.[11]

The distinguishing attribute for the value-based levers is that <u>all the levers are focused on the consumer/patient</u>— they are focused on modifying the consumer behavior to improve health, reduce waste, and deliver quality outcomes. The levers can be used for better adherence to lifestyle management, active participation in a chronic disease management program, adherence to a chronic medication, or use of appropriate health services to obtain the best outcome. The cost is not at the center of the format—cost has been the traditional focal point and experience has shown that putting cost at the center has not contained the costs; they have continued to escalate. With the focus on the person/population, a series or suite of levers will support the behaviors that will drive down the cost trend over time. Keep this in mind: Value-based designs are person-centric. The person, the people, the population that needs to shift to improved management is at the center.

7.1   Tuners Begin with the Beat

The first step in moderating the risk is to have enough data to identify the groups of people who are showing the current risk or are liable to increase risks in the near future. If the company has not installed a health risk appraisal or some way of measuring the current health risks of the population, this is the first place to install a lever. The pace at which you proceed—the "beat"—is determined by the data as this will show you the immediacy of the need, determining how much emphasis you give to each lever and engaging the consumer.

Some companies install a benefit design entry point that causes change: Take the health risk appraisal or insurance benefits will be denied (said in a positive tone: Take the health risk appraisal and we will guide you to enrollment in the benefits plan). While this may seem harsh, as companies grapple with the economic fluctuations, this lever is actually becoming more prominent. Other companies use more of a carrot approach: Take the health risk appraisal and we will deposit money in your health savings account, hold your insurance premium contribution steady with last year's (we will not increase your insurance premium), or we will give you a reward of …(cash, T-shirt, etc.). Each company must decide if the health risk data should include the spouse or dependents, and some companies add an incremental incentive at this point. The incentive must be big enough to get the consumer's attention, and the culture must be secure enough that the employee does not feel he or she may lose her job by disclosing this information. To overcome this fear, many companies use independent third parties and secure website addresses to obtain the data—the company needs the aggregate data for review of population risk, not the person-level data.

The next place a lever can be inserted is to obtain biometric data, such as waist measure, body mass index, blood pressure, cholesterol, glucose and other screenings. Some include depression or stress screenings and some include functional impact (do you have limitations on your ability to perform your job, back pain, etc?), absenteeism, and presenteeism. This section may include prevention and wellness exams, age and gender-appropriate screens (prostate, mammography, colorectal screens). Studies have shown that between 30–60% of a population may have hypertension (high blood pressure) or early stages of diabetes and not even know it.

Using Levers to Engage Consumers and Lower Risk

- **Carrot:** incentive for completion; admission to benefits plan

- **Stick:** Increase in employee insurance contribution; denial of benefits

Behaviors motivated by these levers might include:
- Completion of health risk appraisal
- Completion of biometric screenings or prevention-wellness exam
- Goal-setting, with and without a personal health record
- Use of a personal health record
- Testing for health literacy

Quantifying Risk and Focusing on Risk Reduction. Many experienced employers view this step as one that is too long on return, even if it is short on the effort for implementation. In fact, accumulating relevant data on the population is one of the most important steps in using levers to fine-tune the population behaviors. Simply put, a benchmark is needed to determine the starting risk, predict the future risk, and to look for opportunities for success in moving to better health management. You have to know where you start to know if you are improving. Further, new research from Riedel, et al has shown that lifestyle risks, including physical activity levels, alcohol use, tobacco use, back pain, weight, stress, depression, and driving risk (non-use of seatbelts) contribute to the overall costs of medical care for an employer. The results were then sub-segmented by industry, age, gender and salary to identify the levels of risk that contribute to the overall costs of medical care for an employer.[12]

The annual cost of productivity loss for each person is equal to on-the-job productivity loss percentage multiplied by total annual compensation, which is the product of hourly compensation times 2,080 hours per year. The results showed that:

- Productivity loss was consistently associated with "at risk" health status for all eight of the health risks assessed (Fig. 1).

- Without controlling for any other factors, the biggest differences in productivity loss were observed for those at risk for back pain, stress, and mental well-being.

    ○ Those at elevated risk for back pain in this study sample reported 13.0% more productivity loss than those at low risk for back pain.

○ Those at risk for mental well-being (i.e. depression) reported 7.4% greater productivity loss than those at low risk.

○ Those at risk for stress reported 4.8% greater productivity loss than their low risk counterparts.

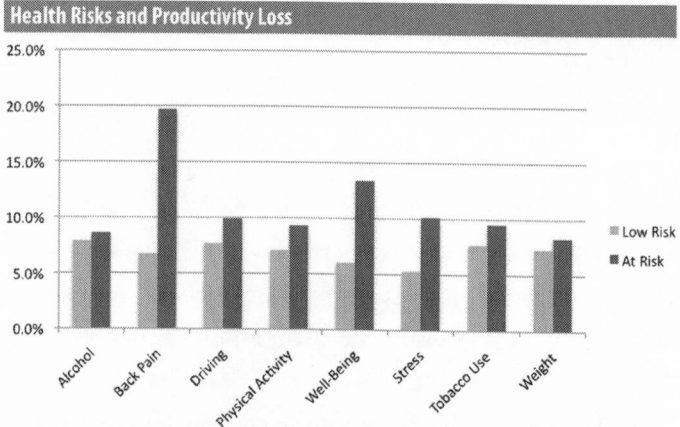

Mean productivity loss for those at low risk and those at risk. All differences were significant based on independent samples t tests. P < 0.001 (Source: Riedel et al, Journal of Occupational and Environmental Medicine)

Although all group differences were statistically significant, these three risk areas represent the greatest potential for meaningful improvement through intervention. The total results were quite stunning, and they support the use of levers to gather population-specific information AND to influence risk reduction as a prime mover for improved population health and corporate health:

- Productivity costs for a person at high risk for all eight factors was 5%, compared with a person at low risk for all eight factors. This 5% higher productivity cost is a significant opportunity for the employer to consider incentives to reduce modifiable risks.

- On average, a person with three health risks cost $5,952 a year in on-the-job productivity loss, a difference of $4,480 when compared with one or no risks, a difference of $1,494 per person.

- Translating this to population health: If 100 people had high-risk for any three of the risk factors measured, and they could reduce just one health risk to low-risk status, this would translate to annual savings of $149,400 (i.e. $1,494 X 100 where the $1,494 is based on the difference in costs for those with three risks v. those with two health risks).

- If 100 individuals moved from three health risks to one, it would yield $298,700 in annual savings.

- If 100 individuals moved from being at risk for three health risks to being at low risk for all eight health risks, it would yield $448,000 in annual savings.

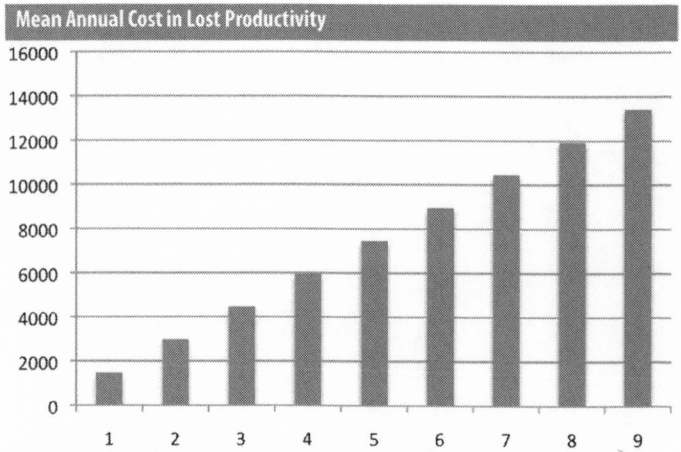

Mean annual cost in lost productivity plotted against the number of health risks for which a person is at risk.
Source: Riedel et al, Journal of Occupational and Environmental Health.

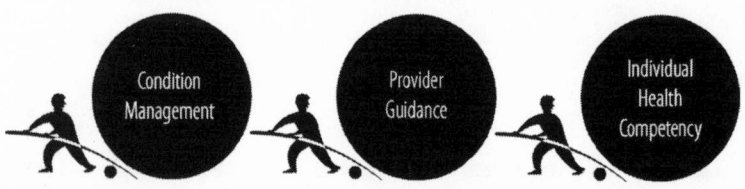

A Champion for Employees

Bill Germanakos, Winner, NBC Season 4 "The Biggest Loser," Director, Corporate Wellness Quest Diagnostics Inc.

Having won the title of "The Biggest Loser" on the NBC hit reality weight loss show of the same name, I now have the unique and rewarding opportunity to act in the capacity of "Wellness Ambassador" for my company, Quest Diagnostics.

In this new position, I truly see the importance of delivering the right messages to employees to engage them in activities such as weight loss programs, smoking cessation programs, or the like.

When employees aren't engaged in company wellness programs, I often see two misperceptions stand in the way of an employee improving his or her own health: 1) they perceive that the company is asking something of them for its own gain, rather than offering something to them as an employee benefit, and 2) they perceive that they are being asked the impossible, because they have tried and failed in the past.

To create an environment where employees are both motivated and empowered to fully engage and take action requires creative and insightful messaging, supported by examples of proven success. In these environments, those who have had success in improving their own health have the opportunity to champion local programs, and even mentor individuals in need of support, and, in turn, help to create more success stories.

As my company's champion of weight loss, I now counsel many of my Quest Diagnostics colleagues who struggle with obesity. They know I've been there, that I can empathize, and can share with them how I myself struggled, what I've learned, and how I finally found my way to overcome my obstacles to losing weight and getting healthy.

A wellness program that seeks out its champions and and puts them in a position to mentor others who are seeking a path to better health not only motivates and inspires colleagues to make a commitment to healthy living, but also motivates that champion to keep the course personally, and show that healthy is indeed a lifestyle. And, I can say from personal experience, that makes it a win - win situation.

7.2   Moderating the Treble: Creating the Memorable Melody or Stickiness

Adherence to behavior change is imperative to the success of trend reduction. There are at least two large buckets that must be considered in order for levers to be designed and implemented:

- What behaviors are inappropriate and driving costs? How does the population (or segment of the population) use services, benefits, and even absenteeism to manage their health, and which of these behaviors need to be modified to a more efficient solution?

- What behaviors do not exist that would be beneficial to the overall health of the population and the organization? Are there segments that get no care at all? How would levers guide them into care that could impact the total health cost trend?

In general, it's a continuous project to move populations to adhere to lifestyle, treatment and services in new behavior patterns. Many employers create designs that improve the stickiness to lifestyle and wellness behaviors. Levers focused on life and health coaching, exercise and nutrition improvement, use of health savings accounts, stress management, and regularly scheduled screenings are often used. As before, these designs may be crafted in the "carrot" approach as well as the "stick" approach.

Employers often look at chronic conditions as a place to begin to improve the stickiness to new behaviors. They believe this is the easiest place to start as it is often the data that is the most "obvious." Levers are inserted that cause people to get their updated exams and labs, to stick with condition management and persistence to treatment, to enroll **and actively participate** in condition management programs, and even to report their activities to the Personal Health Record [PHR] for goal-setting.

Some plan sponsors historically would use enrollment in a condition management program as the primary lever. They saw this as the first step to consumer engagement. Over time, more employers began "pushing the needle," aligning the co-pay reduction lever with active participation in the condition management program. The market continues to gain knowledge and improve, and the experienced plan sponsors have moved into a more sophisticated phase of condition management levers. They now use a suite of levers to engage the consumer in active participation in condition management programs, adherence to treatment and exams, use of medications and recommended testing and goal-setting to reduce risks such as blood sugar control, cholesterol control and blood pressure control.

The often-missed opportunity for stickiness to health management is the group of consumers who have not engaged in healthcare use at all. These folks do not appear in the claims data, and they are not actively managing their health. The employer can review claims data and sub-segment by age, gender, and zip code, as an example, if this data is available. Health Risk Appraisal data may also reveal the age/gender/geographic and even salary bands of populations that are not getting annual wellness exams or not adhering to the chronic care necessary to manage conditions.

Levers to Improve Adherence and Persistence in Condition Management

- **Carrot:** reduction in member costs for access, treatment, or in return for use of PHR/coaching and goal-setting

- **Stick:** increase out-of-pocket costs for insurance benefit, portions of treatments, etc.

Behaviors motivated by these levers might include:
- HSA deposit or incentive for use of Personal Health Record or life coaching
- Reduce co-pays for treatments for defined conditions (such as diabetes, asthma, hypertension, high cholesterol, heart disease, arthritis, depression)
- Reduced insurance premiums if enrolled in lifestyle coaching or condition management
- Increased insurance premiums or co-pays if the person does not engage or drops out of condition management (disease management)

7.3   A Symphony of Performers: Creating a Chorus of Providers

When the person or the population is the focus, then it becomes incredibly important to make sure that communications with valued influencers are effective and efficient. Providers, often the physician or staff, or the pharmacist or staff, provide trusted information that can launch and secure the very behavior change that the plan sponsor is seeking. Therefore, identifying the appropriate levers that will engage the provider networks to support the desired changes is the third "dial" on the tuning scale, or the third concept in levers.

Prevention and wellness exams most often happen through a physician/clinician interaction at the office, through onsite services (clinic, mammography van, hearing and vision screenings), through convenient care clinics and urgent care clinics, over the phone (outbound consultations and telemedicine), and on the Web (e-visits, among others). All of the service providers who touch the consumer must know the health status, the changes in behaviors recommended and completed, and the counseling that has taken place with other providers. A communication platform that links all of these members of the chorus is important, so that they are, literally, all singing from the same hymnal.

If the data shows that there are pockets within the population that use the emergency department as the primary care clinic, then a lever can be installed that causes greater out-of-pocket expense to the consumer. Additionally, a lever can be installed that reduces the out-of-pocket expense for an urgent care or convenient care clinic.

If there are physicians who are getting better results in delivering health (measured according to nationally accepted guidelines, for example), then a co-pay reduction to use these physicians can be used. To align the incentives so that the physician is a willing partner, the employer can also use an incentive that rewards the physician for the time spent to manage the consumer or do the testing based upon the process and outcomes measures of national guidelines—this will often ensure that the connection is made.

Levers to Engage Consumers and Providers in Improved Outcomes

- **Carrot:** reduction in member costs for access, treatment, or for the use of urgent care clinics, convenient care clinics, and onsite services

- **Stick:** increase out-of-pocket costs for emergency room visits

Behaviors motivated by these levers might include:
- Use of the evidence-based guideline physician
- For physician, rewarding taking the time to manage the patient according to evidence-based guidelines
- Use of phone consultations, urgent care clinics, or convenient care clinics
- Use of onsite services and screenings
- Use of in-network providers

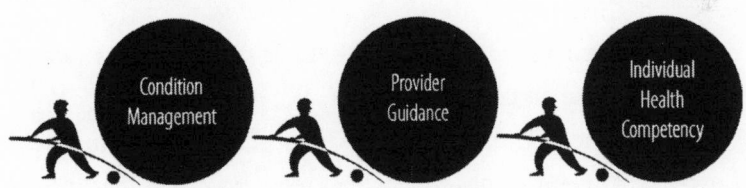

Using the Suite of Levers: Gulfstream Aerospace
A multi-lever approach to consumer engagement[13]

Bob Holben, Director, Global Total Rewards and International Human Resources, Gulfstream Aerospace, and Member of the Board of Directors, Center for Health Value Innovation.

In 2003, Gulfstream Aerospace was in the process of developing its health and wellness strategy for 2004 and beyond. Gulfstream, like most other companies at that time, was experiencing dramatic increases to its medical and pharmaceutical costs. Both of these were trending at double digit rates and the healthcare industry was indicating that, over the next several years, healthcare costs were expected to continue to increase anywhere from 8% to 14%. This would mean that Gulfstream's current healthcare cost would double in five to nine years, something that Gulfstream fully intended to mitigate, or at least delay as much as possible.

While researching possible solutions, Gulfstream's benefits management team encountered a 2001 Institute of Medicine (IOM) paper entitled "Crossing the Quality Chasm" that seemed to offer a major cost-savings opportunity. This report indicated that there was so much waste in the U.S. medical system due to medical and administrative errors that as much as 30% of all medical costs could be attributed to poor quality. This wasted value was totally unacceptable to Gulfstream. As a manufacturer with extremely high quality standards, Gulfstream saw a great opportunity to reduce its healthcare costs through the application of quality control measures within the medical community and by providing oversight to the standards of the healthcare being delivered by the medical community to Gulfstream's employees and their families.

Gulfstream issued an RFP to the two major hospital systems in the Savannah area that specifically asked them to respond to the question of what each hospital system was going to do about the quality of the healthcare being delivered by its hospital and by its network of family care physicians. Gulfstream's current provider, Memorial University Medical Center, delivered the most cost-effective RFP and indicated that it was currently involved with quality improvement initiatives within its hospital system, to include participating in the Medicare/Medicaid CMS initiative. As a result, they were awarded the Gulfstream contract for the next five years. However, Gulfstream's benefits management team insisted that Memorial work with Gulfstream to help design a quality improvement initiative for Memorial's network of primary care physicians who were providing healthcare to Gulfstream's employees and covered dependents. Not only did Memorial agree to work with Gulfstream on that project, but, faced with the business case of reducing their own healthcare costs by up to 30%, they also decided to join with Gulfstream and include their own employees in the program.

Two additional Savannah companies, the Savannah College of Arts and Design (SCAD) and Thomas Hutton Engineering joined the coalition and together they designed and implemented a program they called "Partners in Quality" (PIQ).

Stakeholder Engagement:

For the Partners in Quality program to work effectively, it was essential that all three partners, the employers, the physicians and the employees/dependents, were committed to, and fully engaged in, the process.

Engaging the Companies:

The participating companies were engaged in an effort to reduce their healthcare costs through quality improvement initiatives. The 30% cost of poor quality statistic provided a major financial incentive for each company's CFO to approve their company's participation in the program. In addition, the companies were concerned with the health of their employees and their family members and the impact that a healthy workforce would have on company productivity and profitability. Addressing employee healthcare issues and related costs would also send a powerful message to the employees and their families that the company truly cared about their personal health and well-being.

Engaging the Physicians:

The network of Primary Care Physicians was already personally committed to providing the best possible care to their patients. They became even more engaged when the companies offered a financial incentive to those physicians who exhibited the use of the best practice, evidence-based medicine protocols when treating patients covered under the health plans of the participating companies. For those physicians who met a certain criteria of quality performance, the participating companies would provide a financial payment equal to 20% of the office visit (E&M) charges filed on behalf of the patients covered by the participating companies' medical plans. The focus of the PIQ program's measurement process became the physician's attention to proper, evidence-based treatment protocols for key disease groups. Working with Memorial Hospital's Physician's Quality Committee, the PIQ incentive design team selected Diabetes, Breast Cancer, Cervical Cancer, and Pharmaceutical Management as the areas that represented high medical costs to the participating companies. In addition to the financial reward, each qualifying physician would be designated a "Distinguished Quality Physician" and received public recognition and a certificate suitable for hanging in his or her office.

Engaging the Employees and Their Dependents:

Recognizing that patients need to be actively involved in managing their own health and lifestyle risks, the participating companies knew that they must engage their employees and their covered dependents and obtain their commitment to the quality improvement effort. Communications were distributed that explained how, by being compliant with their physician's treatment orders, employees could save significant amounts of money on healthcare costs for themselves and their families. At Gulfstream, a program was established such that if the employees were compliant with their physician's orders resulting in their doctor becoming recognized as a "Distinguished Quality Physician (DQP)", the employee and their dependents would receive a $5 discount in their office visit co-pays every time they visited that doctor or any other "DQP" physician during the following year [this is a 33% reduction in co-pay]. The employees now had a financial incentive to be responsive to their doctor's orders.

Gulfstream and its Savannah colleagues/employers conducted a major employee communications campaign on that topic of appropriate health resource use. Gulfstream initiated its co-pay reduction program for employees and families who were compliant with their doctors enabling them to become "Distinguished Quality Physicians." The physicians were appreciative *of Gulfstream's efforts and the physician complaints about "non-compliant" patients subsided.*

One other issue the physicians mentioned was that they didn't see the goal of an increased use of generic drugs to be a true measure of the quality of their performance. The employers explained the purpose of that initiative was directly associated with providing patients with cost-effective drug therapies which could also be directly connected with patient compliance. This one measure also had the ability to greatly impact the cost savings and the required return on investment aspect of the entire program.

Almost immediately, this initiative delivered savings to both Gulfstream and its employees. From 2004 to 2007, Gulfstream's generic dispensing rate increased by an additional 24%, going from 33% to 57%, an overall improvement of 73%. The drug industry's "rule of thumb" for generic utilization is that for every one percent increase in a company's generic dispensing rate (GDR), the company could expect an approximate one percent decrease in the company's total annual pharmaceutical cost. Gulfstream has redirected much of these savings back to its employees and their dependents in the form of zero co-pay generic drugs for the treatment of certain chronic diseases and conditions such as asthma, diabetes, high cholesterol, and high blood pressure. In 2009, Gulfstream has expanded its free generic drug program to include generic drugs to treat anxiety and depression. The strat-

egy is that the proper use of drug therapies should greatly impact the health of employees by effectively managing certain illnesses and preventing or delaying certain chronic disease co-morbidities from occurring in others. This would ultimately decrease long-term healthcare costs and improve the company's productivity. The use of free drugs to prevent disease and reduce absences from work was also apparent as Gulfstream conducted its on-site free flu shot program over the past two years. The first year saw 1,424 employees taking part in the program, while participation in the second year increased by 84% to 2,620 employees.

Working with its parent company, General Dynamics, Gulf-stream introduced an Integrated Health Management (IHM) strategy to better coordinate and manage employee absence, medical, disability and workers compensation programs. Implemented through a collaborative effort by both Gulfstream's Benefits and Environmental Health and Safety departments, the primary objective of the IHM initiative was, once again, to reduce all health-related costs while improving the quality of care and overall health status of Gulfstream's employees and their dependents. The IHM program was branded by Gulf-stream as "Partners 2 Health" (P2H). This companywide initiative essentially formed a partnership between Gulfstream and its employees focused on improving the health of all employees and their families, and thereby increasing the productivity and profitability of the total organization. Integral to the P2H process is the challenge of helping employees and their families fully understand their personal responsibility to manage their own health and lifestyle risks. Gulfstream's role is to provide its employees with significant support through comprehensive and creative benefit coverage and robust healthcare resources. "Partners 2 Health" has now become the over-arching program for all Gulfstream wellness initiatives.

Overall Results at Gulfstream

From 2004 through 2007, the impact of the "Partners in Quality" and the "Partners 2 Health" programs were as follows:

- The percent of primary care physicians qualified as "Distinguished Quality Physicians" went from 10% to 44%; an additional 34%, which represents a 340% quality improvement. (18 to 80 doctors)

- The percent of women age 40 and above receiving annual mammograms went from 44% to 51%: reflecting a quality improvement of 16%.

- The percent of diabetics getting two or more HbA1c tests per year went from 39% to 61%; reflecting a 56% quality improvement.

- The percentage of diabetics getting an annual lipid profile went from 57% to 80%; reflecting a 40% quality improvement.

- *The percentage of diabetics who received an annual dilated pupil eye exam went from 32% to 56%; reflecting a 75% quality improvement.*

- *The percentage of women age 21 and above receiving an annual PAP test went from 37% to 63%; reflecting a 70% quality improvement.*

- *The generic drug dispensing rate went from 33% to 54%: reflecting a 64% quality improvement.*

- *There was a 21% reduction in average medical cost per diabetic.*

- *There was a 2% reduction in diabetic patients with renal failure.*

- *There was a 43.3% increase in average drug cost per diabetic. (This is a good thing! These added drug therapies help eliminate or delay diabetic co-morbidities.)*

- *Gulfstream's four year healthcare cost increase trend was only 4.3%.*

- *Gulfstream's programs have generated an annual healthcare cost avoidance of $5 to $6 million.*

Chapter 8

REAL-WORLD BUSINESS RESULTS WITH SUITES OF LEVERS

"If you build it, they will not come, unless incented.

For many years, I believed that the desire for improved health would drive most people to change unhealthy aspects of their lifestyle, if only given the right tools. Unfortunately my experience has shown me that this is not the case. Other levers must be used such as value driven benefit design and direct incentives."

ROBERT SCULLY, MD
SENIOR MEDICAL DIRECTOR
HEALTH ALLIANCE MEDICAL PLANS

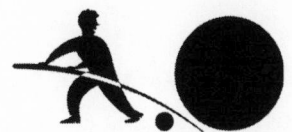

Levers can be used in a myriad of combinations to affect the outcome of improved health and reduced financial trend for both the person and the organization. In this chapter there are several overviews of the impact of levers, through benefits designs, incentives and disincentives that cause the desired behavior change.

For a level setting, the following are the key points of the iconic experiences of both Pitney Bowes and Asheville, North Carolina.

8.1   Pitney Bowes[14]

For many years, Pitney's health costs were competitive with benchmark results that were trending at low single-digit rates. This situation changed in the late 1990s. Because Pitney already had 10 years of experience in gathering and integrating data and applying the learnings to influence employee behavior, it was well-suited to move into the value-based design launch in late 2001.

In the early 1990s, Pitney began by creating a totally integrated data warehouse that assembled data on medical claims, disability, workers' compensation, job band/zip/, and other demographics utilization of on-site medical clinics . This data base could be mined to show key cost drivers, influencers and ultimately predictors for high cost claims.

- *LEVER: Create a recognized network of clinicians and incentive to guide employees to their use.* Pitney developed guidelines for purchasing and aligned the incentives to steer *utilization* to those providers who delivered high quality, efficient care.

- *LEVER: Create an incentive to improve personal/individual health management.* Pitney developed Healthcare University *in* the early 1990s, incentivizing employees to learn to about their lifestyles, chronic care, and health management, and to adopt or maintain those health behaviors that support improved functional health.

- *LEVER: Remove cost barriers to appropriate care in the highest cost-driving conditions.* In 1995, Pitney tested the concept of lowering access to behavioral health (which was the standard at the time) and studying the result: Higher behavioral costs as well as medical claims in the affected population.[15] This approach was dropped in 1997 when Pitney Bowes moved to full parity for mental health and substance abuse treatment including a free eight-session EAP model.

When the call-to-action came in late 1999 to address costs, Pitney Bowes decided to take a pro-active approach. There was enough of a culture of health as well as data integration to make giant leaps into new territory: The use of levers to change risky behaviors, including lack of care, misuse of care, and under-use of care. Their data showed that pharmaceutical compliance for several chronic diseases was not compatible with optimal results.[16]

- *LEVER: The suite of levers to remove access barriers—costs to maintaining the treatment—were installed to increase the use of appropriate treatment: All medications used to treat hypertension, asthma and diabetes were moved to 1st tier 10% co-insurance, prevention and wellness exams were pre-deductible (little or no cost).*

The results: A modest increase in total pharmaceutical costs, but a dramatic decrease in the trend for the target chronic medical conditions. Over the years, this plan has been modified to include, for example, waived co-pays for statin medications for high-risk populations (those with a cardiac event or diagnosed diabetes). In the first five years of installation, generic fill rates rose, all medication possession ratios approached 80% (meaning that 80% of the yearly number of prescribed medications were filled). Since inception to 2007, the average annual increase, on a per employee basis, has been 6.8%.

The Pitney Bowes Timeline

More than 18 years of innovation using plan design to change behavior

DATA warehouse	Exclusive Provder Org, Health Care University	EAP – Behavioral Health	Predictive models developed: "Who will cost $10,000 or more in the next 35 years?"	Value-based benefits launch	Costs start to decline	First "free" Rx design for high-risk populations
1990	1993-94	1995	1997-99	2001	2002	2007

© 2009 Center for Health Value Innovation

It's important to remember that this has been, and is continuing to be, an 18-year journey of installing a culture of health, rewarding the appropriate behaviors, reducing barriers to care, promoting the results, and re-thinking the latest data for performance improvement.

8.2 Asheville, North Carolina

The story of lever-driven and value-based design in Asheville is one of two employers, the City of Asheville and Mission St. Joseph's Hospital, coming together to efficiently control the diabetes epidemic. They, too, removed access barriers to appropriate care, but in order to get the care with the waived co-pay, the patient had to be part of a condition-management program. This, then, was fundamentally different from the Pitney suite of levers.

In Asheville, diagnosed patients with diabetes were offered the following:

- *LEVER: Mandatory involvement in condition management program.* Patients were encouraged to enroll in a diabetes management program that involved meeting with the pharmacy counselor and the diabetes educator on a prescribed schedule. If the patient did not do this, the entire cost of care was charged to him/her.

- *LEVER: Access barriers removed by waiving the costs of total treatment.* With enrollment, the patient received waived co-pays for prescription medication, labs, exams, counseling visits.

Results: 35% decrease in direct healthcare spend (medical claims, pharmacy claims, labs, inpatient days, emergency room visits); HbA1C decrease of 6% (HbA1C is a measure of diabetes management success); 50% decrease in absenteeism; savings ~$500 per employee.[17]

These are the brief overviews of the earliest implementers of value-based designs using levers to drive desired behaviors, measuring results, then adjusting the levers to fine-tune the performance. In no way are these two iconic models in value-based design the total story—they are a part of the story in which innovators used the four-step value-based design process to achieve their goals:

- **Data** to determine risk and opportunity,

- **Design** through benefit and incentives, with suites of levers, to influence desired behaviors,

- **Delivery** of services and communications linking incentives across the stakeholders to drive sticky behavior change, and

- **Dividends** in the form of both direct and indirect desired results.

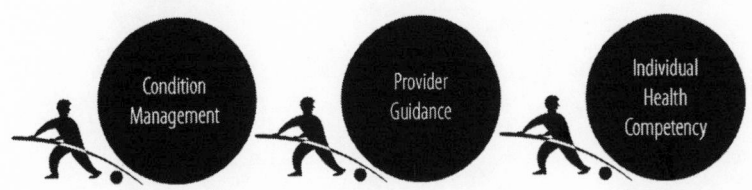

Kavita V. Nair, Ph.D, Associate Professor, School of Pharmacy, University of Colorado Denver

Merely providing financial incentives to improve patient adherence for prescription medications is limiting. Adherence is a complex phenomenon that should be the combined responsibility of the patient and their provider. VBBD efforts that are aimed at improving adherence should consider the dual role of patients and providers in designing incentives to improve adherence.

Chapter 9

LEARNING TO DRIVE THE VALUE USING THE LEVERS

"One size does not fit all. The most important aspect of value-based design is reviewing the customer's member population and understanding the main health issues. From there, we can offer a customized approach—a suite of tools — that employers can use with a variety of benefit design options that will encourage engagement, promote wellness and establish health improvement."

BRIAN SWEET, B.S. PHARM, M.B.A.
CHIEF PHARMACY OFFICER
WELLPOINT, INC.

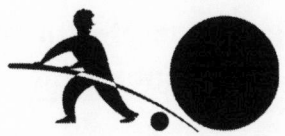

Levers can be implemented through the insurance design (adjusting co-pays and co-insurance levels, moderating out-of-pocket expenses, requiring participation in disease or condition management programs, accessing prevention and wellness exams through a pre-deductible status or Health Savings Account contribution). Levers can also be used as stand-alone incentives or disincentives that create the desired behavior change.

The following three overviews show the impact of using levers to performance-tune the behaviors of your population. In each case, the total story is compacted for ease of learning—there is always more data that was considered, more stakeholder involvement (getting the CEO-CFO to "buy in" to the idea), more communication linking all of the providers into a seamless system around the patient(s). These high-level snapshots are included here so that the use of multiple levers in many settings can be studied and then translated to other situations and evidence.

9.1   Improving Individual Health, from the Detroit Chamber Regional Chamber

In a situation where small, fully-insured employers partnered with their health plan (therefore, only aggregate data was made available by the carrier) the use of the Health Risk Appraisal, Biometric Screen, Goal Setting and Aligned Benefit Incentives drove outcomes that showed positive results. Employee behavior drives the benefit level, so access to enhanced benefits are a result of appropriate behavior. The insurance premium charged for the enhanced level was lower than if the employer purchased it outright, and only one premium was charged regardless of whether a subscriber qualified for enhanced or standard benefits.

- *LEVER: Mandatory health risk appraisal and biometric screen drive enriched benefit access.* The Health Risk Appraisal and correlated Biometric Screen were used to accumulate enough data on the current and predicted risk of the population. The enrollee who took both had a richer benefit offering than those people who did not participate.

- *LEVER: Goal setting for improved health competency.* Outcomes at the person-level were communicated to each enrollee, and the enrollee set his/her goal for health improvement for the year. Points were established that qualified the person for enriched benefits, including lower co-pays for physician visits, treatments, etc.

The following chart shows some of the results from the use of these levers[18]:

Results from Use of Health Levers

# Identifid as At Risk	Measure Applied	Agreement to Improve	Percentage of Eligible Adults	Estimated Medical Loss Ratio
1,722	Agreed to quit smoking	1,616	7.6%	110-140%
	Enrolled in Quit the Nic* (n=1,616)	1,164	72% of those who agreed to quit	
6,321	Agreed to control weight	5,772	28%	110-140%
1,544	Agreed to control blood pressure	1,524	6.5%	120-150%
5,477	Agreed to control cholesterol	5,347	23%	100-130%
1,393	Agreed to control blood sugar	1,342	5.7%	125-150%
211	Agreed to control alcohol use	159	0.6%	125-150%
Number asked to return to their primary care physicians for follow-up		8,778	37.7%	

Overall, the effort to engage the person in the management of individual health resulted in improved health status for the participant and a dividend up to 150% to the employer/payer, reflected in the medical loss ratio estimations.

9.2 Improving Status through the Guidance to Care Providers

QuadMed, a wholly owned subsidiary of Quad/Graphics, is a primary-care medical home that provides onsite services to its employees and their dependents. It is also a successful brand that is franchised to other companies because of its success in managing multiple levers for year-over-year trend rates of 4.7% and below.

The philosophy and culture of QuadMed and Quad/Graphics is one of family and inclusion. The family-owned business is self-insured, founded by the Quadracci family in Wisconsin, and considers its employees and their families as part of the larger family of the organization. They have a Culture of Health in which access barriers are reduced for appropriate care, physicians are rewarded for the outcomes and care provided (rather than the numbers of patients that can be crammed into an hour), electronic medical records are the norm, and evidence-based guidelines are the standard.

QuadMed found that, with increasing body mass index (BMI), the costs of care for people who had BMI over 27.1 (overweight or obese) escalated to the following indicators:

- 82% higher use of pharmaceutical drugs;

- 80% higher inpatient days;

- 78% higher outpatient days.

Levers were installed to flatten this escalation in cost as well as reduce the health risks of the population.

- *LEVER: Mandatory health risk appraisal and Biometric Screen.* The use of the HRA and Biometric Screen provided onsite, and at no cost to the participant, is the gateway to benefits.

- *LEVER: Enrollment in condition management is required for enriched benefits.* Comprehensive condition management includes:

  o obesity and weight management for those at risk for obesity;

  o required health coaching and diabetes educators for those diagnosed with diabetes, which leads to waived co-pays for physician exams, labs, and treatments/ medications;

  o required enrollment in smoking cessation classes leading to waived co-pays for many stop-smoking treatments.

- *LEVER: Incentives for physicians to treat the chronic care patients.* Physicians are part of the incentive-based design. They treat the population with evidence-based guidelines, and they are rewarded for the time and outcomes, rather than for the number of patients they see in one day. This creates a win in the physician community, as each physician uses his/her total skill set and complete treatment team to achieve the best outcome for the patient and the family, including QuadMed-Quad/Graphics.

- *LEVER: Waived co-pay for the use of onsite services.* Because QuadMed is located onsite with rich services and complete coaching, there is an incentive for the patient to use the onsite services for all of his or her primary and workers' compensation needs.

This is the total alignment of incentives for provider guidance—creating the lever to drive the patients to the preferred provider group AND creating the incentive for the provider to treat the patient in the manner that produces the best outcomes for both the patient and the payer/employer. The results are impressive: In this Mercer actuarial accounting, QuadMed consistently surpasses the rates of inflation for benchmarked companies as well as the national norms for health costs per member per year—by over 30%.

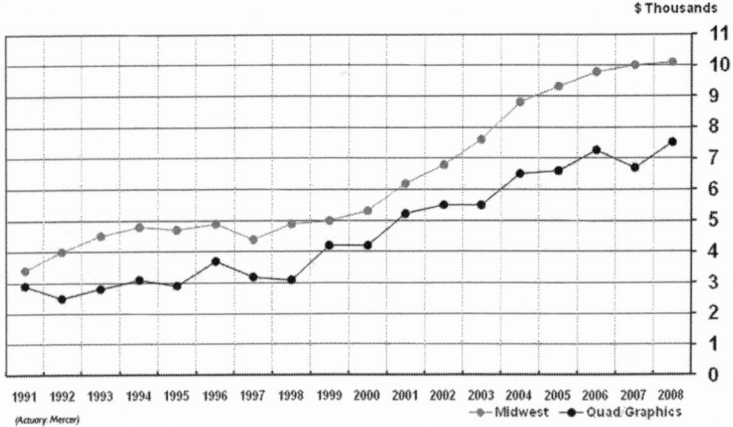

This graph shows a consistent 4.9% trend year over year for approximately 11,000 members, with an actual decrease in total health costs for year 2007. These are net figures; all costs are loaded into the graph.

"My boss – Joel Quadracci, CEO of Quad/Graphics – has become fond of asking the rhetorical question in executive forums, 'Who would've ever thought that health care would turn out to be a competitive advantage for a printing company?' It is precisely because of our Value-Based Benefit Design that Joel can put forth that bold assertion. The combination of VBID, coupled with our personalized, proactive approach to primary care delivered at our on-site 'medical home' clinics allows us to enjoy significant cost savings AND demonstrably better measures of population health."

Raymond J. Zastrow, M.D., FAAFP
President, QuadMed

9.3   Improving Outcomes through a Focus on Condition Management

The iconic experiences of Pitney Bowes and Asheville NC are two examples of chronic condition management, although it's important to remember they also included individual health improvement as well as provider guidance, where appropriate. But there are many examples of the use of levers to drive improved condition management, pushing related unhealthy conditions and costs into the future. One of these examples is the use of levers in a county in the southeast United States.

Since 2005, Mike Kushner, the Risk Manager of the self-insured Polk County, Florida, has used a suite of levers to manage those with diagnosed diabetes and hypertension (high blood pressure). The suite of levers identifies those at risk through a health risk appraisal and Biometric Screen plus integration of data to the claims data. From there, the levers are designed to keep the diagnosed members persistent with their prescribed treatment.

- *LEVER: Incentives for enrollment in the coaching and condition management programs.* Members who are diagnosed with diabetes and hypertension are encouraged to "opt in" to the management programs offered, and are then given access to richer benefits to manage their conditions.

- *LEVER: Incentives for treatment keep persistency high.* Members who actively participate in the condition management program, receiving timely exams, labs, and refills, get their treatment at incentive levels. If the rules of participation are not followed, the participant is given two strikes and then is dis-enrolled from the program. Actively enrolled participants are provided the benefit of $0 co-pays for medication and supplies related to their diabetes or hypertension.

- *LEVER: Contract for goal-setting ensures compliance with treatment recommendations.* Active participants must set a contractual goal with their health coach in order to be considered an "active" member in the program and receive their treatments at waived co-pay levels.

The results are impressive: Medication possession ratios, the indicator of the right amount of refills and, therefore, the adherence levels to recommended treatment, improved. Twenty-two percent (22%) of diabetes participants in the highest severity stratification changed to a lower severity stratification. The reduction of HbA1C (a measure of successful diabetes control) was noted in the diabetic population, most notably in the highest-risk diabetes patients. Reduction in blood pressure in hypertension patients, particularly those who were classified as having the highest severity, was also recorded.

The reduction in non-adherence, the improvement in health status indicators, and the improvement in health competency all contributed to the overall reduction in financial trend for this self-insured county representing 900 lives.

9.4 Real-World Evidence across Business Sectors, Sizes and Geographic Areas

In the 80+ interviews and over 150 online surveys conducted by the Center, the group of levers and sophistication in the suites has grown. Different levers are used by each company, whether large manufacturer, small city, or health system as an employer, as the culture and data indicate. The numbers of people who are not receiving any care, who are diagnosed with conditions but are not following evidence-based guidelines, or who are choosing highly expensive interventions such as emergency department visits for primary care—these are key indicators of priorities for design change that can reduce risk, improve health management, and guide folks to appropriate care. As a summary, the levers influence the activities the plan sponsor wants to improve. The following chart shows the macro-levers, the rolled up plan designs and incentives that have shown to deliver quality outcomes and reduce financial trend.[19]

15 Levers Across 3 Categories

Individual health— Prevention-Wellness
- Insurance premium or benefit cost held stable for completion or participation in HRA, biometric screen, prevention exam or Personal Health Record (PHR) use
- Mandatory health risk appraisal with incentive (co-pay reduction, HSA deposit)
- Health promotion goal: OOP reduced by setting and/or achieving goal
- Prevention : yearly exam cost is waived, paid 100%, or is considered pre-deductible
- Prevention: age-gender appropriate screen/inoculations waived or lowered co-pay or co-insurance (such as flu shots, mammograms, prostate screens, colonoscopy, etc)
- Business channel incentives: all members of a business channel or team, or the head of the business channel alone, are incentivized to achieve process goals of personal health mgt as part of their yearly business objectives

Care management
- Lifestyle coaching is mandatory
- Generics are lowered to a $0-10 co-pay
- Condition-based formulary is adjusted (all tiers are lowered for specified condition/s)
- Mandatory condition management linked to co-pay/co-insurance waivers (enroll in the classes/phone calls, etc., and the total cost of care is reduced or waived)
- Prior authorization, step tiering, etc. for low-value treatments (this is part of the incentive-disincentive mix, where some costs for treatments or drugs are raised in order to steer consumers away from lower-value interventions, or to put more out of pocket costs on the consumer—thereby reducing total costs to the plan sponsor—so that total health care costs remain at or close to neutral.)

Care Delivery
- Reduced-waived co-pay or HSA deposit for use of providers w evidence-based and patient-centered practices
- Aligned reimbursement to providers for practice change/improvement
- Reduced-waived co-pay for destination (onsite, medical travel, phone-web consultations, urgent care clinic, etc)
- Increased OOP expense for use of non-preferred destination-provider (ER, multi-MRI, etc)

9.5   Comparative information

Sometimes, it's helpful to see comparative results in one chart. The following graph showcases additional self-reported results from the database of the Center for Health Value Innovation. In each case, the employer or payer was asked:

- What was your health cost trend year over year from 2005-2008?

- What designs of incentives/disincentives did you use, within or outside your benefit structure?

- What results did you see, and, where available, please report on a PMPM (per member per month) or PMPY (per member per year) level for comparison.

Company	Levers	Benefit Design	Results
		Using Levers for Performance	
A	C	• Diabetes management with educator required for waived co-pays • Cost to payer of about $400 pppy	• 50% of group also received pharmacy consultation. This group saved 21% on unscheduled absences.
B	I, P, C	• Generic statins at $0 co-pay • Focus on cardiovascular disease and diabetes	• January '06-'07, number of heart attack hospital claims down 55% • Savings of $750,000 per month at employer level, $175,000 at member level
C	P, C	• Lower co-pays for generic ($4) and branded ($15%) drugs for diabetes • Mandatory diabetes educator visits • Custom molded shoe inserts for diabetics • Preferred Provider tiering using evidence-based guidelines • No limits on smoking cessation benefits	• Total cost reduced 27%, about $1,306 pmpy • 50% of patients with high blood pressure at goal (130/80) or improving • 84.3% of patients measured were at goal for cholesterol (<200) • 51.6% at goal of HbA1c under 7.0 • Condition awareness up from 2.83 to 4.31 at post-assessment
D	C	• Colorectal screenings • Smoking cessation program	• Saved $5 million in absenteeism and productivity loss • Net claims savings of more than $1 million due to early detection • $1 million net savings in 3 years

Levers: I= Individual Health, P=Provider Selection, C=Condition Management

The key messages for using levers for performance tuning or, in benefits and incentive design to drive the value of health dollars spent, are:

- **Data drives decisions.** Accumulate as much as you can, and begin to develop relational information by ages, genders, salaries, geographies, etc.

- **Design drives behavior change.** Consider the behaviors that would improve the value of every dollar spent.

What are you purchasing—is it the number of touches in a condition management program or the improved health that could result?

- **Delivery is dependent upon the health management skills** of the population you wish to affect. How are you creating opportunities and amplifying success in skill development? Are there coordinated communication links so that the physician, the patient and the condition management people are aligned in the goals and the treatment progression? Is the environment in sync with the goals you are trying to accomplish? Are there healthy foods in vending machines, flex time for physician appointments, and even stress breaks throughout the day? Are you communicating often enough? Is access close enough or can it be improved and enhanced?

- **Dividends are a result of the behavior changes,** so align the incentives and disincentives to achieve the desired outcomes (consequences). Anticipate the unintended consequences that could happen.

Create a committee across various business channels in your company; some of these people should not be related to health and safety outcomes. Let these representatives from across the company test your ideas in order to minimize the unintended consequences of the design changes. When considering the levers, make sure to use them to stimulate the activity that will drive the results intended: Active, healthy, productive members of the business or community.

Chapter 10

ECONOMIC SECURITY IS TIED TO COMMUNITY HEALTH AND INNOVATION

"We are at a unique crossroads. We can continue to pay the system for units of care, and we will receive what we always have: Higher costs per unit and struggling economies. Or we can create communities of health where we pay for units of health, and we will get healthier people, healthier businesses, and healthier bottom lines."

PETER HAYES
DIRECTOR OF ASSOCIATE HEALTH AND WELLNESS
HANNAFORD SUPERMARKETS

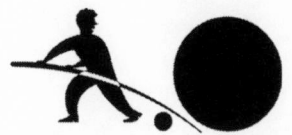

The road to improved health outcomes is paved with the learnings and challenges shared by those who came before. The Health Value Continuum—the entrants, champions, fast followers and renegades who began the early innovations and taught them to others—has grown and morphed into a very defined journey of improving individual health, provider selection and/or chronic condition management. By removing waste from the system (getting the annual exam but not the Biometric Screens, filling the first prescription for a condition but not filling the remainder, using the emergency department as a primary care clinic) and increasing efficiencies (self-management of health and conditions, appropriate use of urgent care and convenient care clinics, for example), the payer as well as the patient/member can achieve healthier outcomes in risk and financial measures.

A review of some popular benefits designs using the levers is captured in the next chart. Remember that this is not an exhaustive list.

Examples of Levers in Benefits Designs and in Incentive Designs

Individual Health	1. Access to information	Co-pay for biometric screens, tests, on-site services, etc. Waiver or reward for coaching, mentoring, business channel improvements	Early steps moderate risk, drive improvement	3 months
	2. Personal context and relevance		Compliance and persistence improved	
	3. Goal-setting	Coaching, peer support, on-time and relevant communication	Culture of health, on-time reinforcement	9-12 months
			All-stakeholder connectivity (safety net is secured)	6-12 months
Chronic Condition Management	1. Access to treatment	Co-pay reductions for treatments (prescriptions and others)	Reduced inpatient and emergency visits	9-18 months
	2. Access to physicians, clinicians	More hours, technology assist	Reduced disability, absenteeism	9-12 months
		Enriched benefits, incentive into health savings account, reward for activity in		6-12 months
	3. Persistency	condition management, etc.	Reduced co-morbidity	months
			Enhanced link to wealth	18-36 months
Provider Guidance	1. Access to diagnosis	Co-pay for biometric screens and tests	Early detection, early treatment, etc.	9-12 months
	2. Access to physician	Guidance, on-site services, more hours, tech assist	Reduction in number and severity of co-morbid conditions	12-24 months
		Enriched benefits for HRA use, PHR use, condition	Improved competency before chronic diagnosis	3-9 months
	3. Persistency	management	Improved competency for total health management	6-9 months

Population health focuses on the **group health indicators** that drive cost, utilization and development of risk/disease. Using levers can drive down the trends in direct costs, over- and under-utilization of services, health risks and financial risks, and exacerbated conditions. Pushing cost and health decrements into the future drive the outcome desired. Improving skills, communication and health management efficiency is the fuel to achieve the end-location: Healthier, more productive workforces, families and communities.

So, what's next?

10.1 Innovators Don't Stop Innovating

With every new design there are new risks uncovered. As innovators share their results, they learn and consider the applications within their own world. This is the very essence of scientific change, and it's no different in the business world.

New innovations are focused on more targeted levers. The emerging science of personalized medicine will create levers that are even more individualized. There are new diagnostic tests and communications that are being developed to more accurately identify, within a population, the people most likely to develop a disease or manage a condition less skillfully. Once identified, a lever or suite of levers will encourage these populations to actively seek help for skill building or switch to more appropriate treatments.

There are emerging tests that will better identify appropriate medications at an individual level. As an example, in the diabetes community, the HbA1C blood test is one test used as a marker for increased risk of diabetes. But new analyses are being developed that can provide a laser focus on who will really develop diabetes—not everyone with higher HbA1C will develop diabetes, and some will develop a condition known as pre-diabetes before HbA1C is elevated. If the new test can accurately identify the most likely sub-segment to develop diabetes, then new interventions that help to push the disease far out into the future can be targeted to those individuals. Imagine that the same number of dollars, differently distributed, can help those most at-risk to change their behaviors and reduce the number of years that they will live with diagnosed diabetes and all its complications. This cost-neutral lever holds promise for both the individual and the payer or employer.

New innovations use existing behaviors to identify those at risk in untraditional ways. Some plan sponsors and payers (health plans) are experimenting with concepts unrelated to health management that may be indicators for poorer health outcomes. Innovators in this category are identifying, through retrospective claims analysis and integration with compensation information, that people who do not contribute to their future health through health savings account, wellness exams, or 401K contributions (for example) also have poorer health outcomes. The hypothesis is that these folks may not be "invested" in the future, and they, again, could be a priority for more intense counseling, health coaching, and reduction in access barriers to teach them health competency.

New innovations use technology to speed improved health skills. When access and communication are linked, the outcomes may go up exponentially. This is being measured through online or telephonic consultations, through the use of digital transmission (such as 24-hour radiology interpretation by using capacity of radiologists in different time zones), personal health records and electronic medical records. Additionally, communities are aggregating health claims and other information in order to track trend in a geographic area so that new levers can influence the health of communities. Even the capacity and efficiency of hospitals and health systems to provide care are now being tracked through technology to guide the patient to the right physician, the right hospital, and the right procedure, when necessary.

New innovations monitor efficiency in remote locations. The concept of medical travel is not new. For decades, Americans have used the services of health systems of excellence for their care—systems such as Mayo, M.D. Anderson, Cleveland Clinic, and many others. The focus now on Medical Tourism, defined as international travel for particular interventions, is one that uses quality measures of safety, improved health, continuity of care, and electronic information transfer to assure global health access around the world. There is a rapid rise in the use of Medical Tourism, or Medical Travel (which may sound a bit less frivolous) within the United States. For those who can plan ahead for testing or elective procedures, Medical Travel can drive efficiency through the competent skills located within another location coupled with the technology to keep the original primary care physician "in the loop" for patient care.

New innovations link outcomes to incentives through contractual arrangements. Some health plans, pharmaceutical companies, medical device companies, and employers are creating new contractual concepts and testing them. The magic in a value-based design is that once the incentives are aligned there is general population health improvement. The degree, acceleration of uptake and measurement of the aligned improvement can be used to create new contracts that focus on the person and the population instead of the number of treatments or the formulary positioning of the drug. Instead of pricing condition management services on the number of patients touched, new contracts are focused on the number of patients who actually improve, and they are sharpened when the time-to-improvement is reduced.

CASE in point: CIGNA and Merck announced on April 26, 2009 that they had entered into a mutual contract that creates rewards for better outcomes, no matter which drug is used. The contract, as reported in the *New York Time[20]s* (and commented upon by members of the Center in other national and regional media), works like this:

- A higher rebate was paid to CIGNA for the placement of Januvia and Janumet, the Merck drugs for diabetes, onto 2nd tier, a better position for the drugs than the previous 3rd tier. NOTE: This is nothing new—it is a standard in the formulary (preferred drug) contracting.

- Rebates on the Merck drugs escalate because they will be used more due to the formulary position of "preferred brand." Again, this is not new.

- Rebates will be escalated AGAIN if the population, REGARDLESS of the drugs used, achieve control of diabetes, defined by reduction in HbA1C levels. This means that Merck and CIGNA are actually partnering on the total improvement of the covered population. As an example, if people who are treated by metformin (a generic first-line intervention for diabetes) reduce their HbA1C levels, then Merck will pay a higher rebate to CIGNA even though the patients were not on the Merck drug and Merck does not manufacture metformin.

This is one of many contracts coming forward in which the PERSON is put at the center of the contract instead of the cost. The OUTCOMES of the population are the key metric, not the use of the drug. The Condition Management expertise at CIGNA is now aligned with the contractual arrangement from Merck, so that both companies will work in tandem to achieve better outcomes and share savings in total health costs with the plan sponsor (employer/payer) and, hopefully, the providers and patients.

To date, by calling for outcomes-based contracting that focuses on person/population health improvement, the Center for Health Value Innovation is creating "buzz" and success in health plans, in employers, and throughout the manufacturing industry, aligning incentives and creating new platforms for collaboration.

10.2 Pushing the Boundaries of Innovation

Some experienced innovators continue to re-think the innovation and value-defined space. When the person is at the focus of the thinking, new ideas develop that begin to broaden the suite of solutions available. Using the concepts of health, wealth, and personal improvement, some innovators are re-shaping the landscape to personalize benefits to meet the member needs. Just as some folks like vanilla or chocolate ice cream, some folks like health savings accounts and some don't; some folks like using preferred provider networks and some don't; some would like personal time off as a reward while others may choose career training as a lever.

It is important to remember that levers are utilized to change a consumer's health behavior to one that is more desirable, and sometimes they are utilized to align behaviors of all stakeholders, such as improved disease management from the health plan or care coordination at the provider level.

This is maximized when the behavior change is tied to personal relevance. The motivating factor for the consumer must tie to the business goals of the plan sponsor, the success of the provider, and the needs of the market overall. By providing choices to the consumer that will accomplish both the person goals and the business goals, aligned improvement can result—these are the dividends that create sustainable behavior change. The sharper the lever or suite of levers to accomplish this goal, the more successful the behavior change, the faster the dividends, and the better improvement for the consumer and the community.

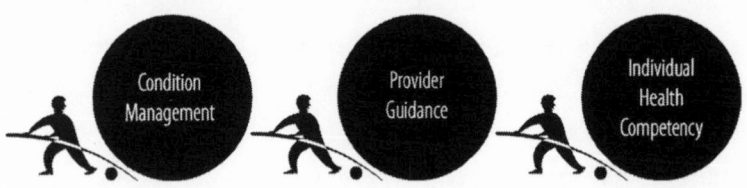

The Voice of an Innovator, Chris McSwain, Vice President of the Center for Health Value Innovation (Chris is an expert in Benefits and Compensation, currently employed at a Fortune 50 company and responsible for global benefits and compensation)

Especially in today's economy, employees are the final differentiator for each employer. Each employee owns his or her health, wealth and career. Health, wealth and career are assets in which both the employer and each employee make investments annually.

Most employers do not track, measure or work to optimize this important annual investment in their employees. For each employer this annual investment in their people can be 10%, 15%, 20% or a higher percentage of annual revenue. Typically, minimal resources are present in Human Resources to really manage these investments, levels that are not similar to what exists in other areas of their business.

For employees, the sum of their health, wealth and career assets reflects their personal value. In other words, Health + Wealth + Career = Personal Value (PV). For employers, the sum of all employees' PV represents the Human Capital of the enterprise. Higher levels of personal accountability for these PV assets drive higher employee engagement levels in employer's programs to improve the Human Capital of the enterprise.

Health, wealth and career are all intrinsically linked - decisions in one area often impact the other two. For example, an employee can't save enough to pay for poor health in retirement. Additionally, poor health leads to diminished productivity and performance, which in turn impacts career potential resulting in lesser wealth over time. Levers improving health always have an impact wealth and career, but most employers are not consciously considering this linkage when managing health and productivity costs.

How can employers, with same or lesser costs, manage their Human Capital assets while increasing value perceived by employees? Personalization of rewards provides the opportunity to meet the present and changing needs of employees through their employment. Personalization of health, wealth and career options at the individual level strengthens the employer's value proposition available for each employee by helping them increase their PV with options that make sense for them. The total benefits and compensation package should be relevant and changeable for each employee so that, throughout the employment and the career of the individual, health, wealth, and career opportunities and success are aligned.

Increased PV results in improved engagement, performance and retention - all key measures for employers. Personalization of health, wealth and career investments provides employers with a strategy to differentiate themselves in the marketplace through their most important asset - their Human Capital.

10.3 Building Communities of Health Value

Expanding the focus from the employer and payer to the community in which they live is the next step for innovation. Communities of Health Value can be developed through the use of the same levers that drove populations of health improvement. Starting with the levers and categories that already exist—individual health, provider guidance, chronic condition management—the influence can be extended to the community level. In this dynamic, the innovative employer assumes a leadership role and assists a multi-stakeholder group in developing a 4th category of lever: Environmental measures that support, insure, and propel improved health.

> "With the globalization of health care and the ease of travel, consumers now have access to care at Centers of Medical Value outside of their local communities. Medical travel, whether it is across the country or overseas, emerges as an alternative option for medical treatment. Going forward, Centers of Medical Value – wherever they are located, both domestic and abroad – are positioned to attract patients who are willing to travel for quality, cost-efficient care. This growing phenomenon will have a significant presence in medical care management."

Laura Carabello, publisher, Medical Travel Today

Communities of Health Value must start with the aligned stakeholders to create a comprehensive "supply chain" focused on total health improvement. These stakeholders could include hospital/health systems, provider organizations or small practices, employers (including governments as employers), community advocacy groups (such as American Heart Association, school boards, etc.). They focus on a collectively-developed set of outcomes that can be achieved in the short term and longer term. Their underpinning is on the reduction of redundancy (overuse in the system, or overbuilding of resources) and efficiency (using evidence and goal-setting to affect the desired change in health behaviors and outcomes) and a shared financial reward for all.

Central to all of this alignment is a culture of health value, in which the environment of safety, health and wealth are linked. The employee/consumer becomes the CEO of his/her health and wealth, and the resulting outcomes feed the value of the community.[21] The Center of Medical Value becomes crucial to the Community, although Centers of Medical Value for certain procedures may exist in neighboring towns or across the country—these are built on competency, experience, safety and medical error reduction, evidence-based guidelines, and a continuity of care that promotes return-to-home and work. The Centers of Medical Value attract the appropriate medical personnel and payments to create sustainability; they attract the needed technology and communication to create persistency; and they connect the health-wealth portfolio of each patient (appropriate services at transparent pricing), payer (efficiency and efficacy), and system level (improved business security because of diminished waste and improved financial trend).

The following diagram shows how the relationships build to develop a Community of Health Value that can create economic security at the community level.

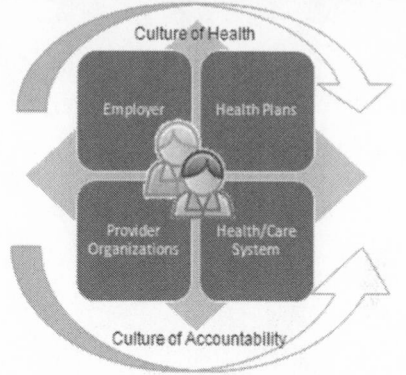

Communities of health value will drive aligned economic advantages so that business that already lives there can thrive, and new business will be attracted, providing new input into the innovation, economic security, and the talent pool available.

As these communities of value grow and mature, greater community penetration and activation can occur. Imagine a community of health value that chooses to create community gardens for greater access to fresh fruits and vegetables or grocery stores that have healthy cooking nights. Bringing all of these activities and a greater number of stakeholders together can bring even greater value and improved outcomes. The result becomes a sustainable economic environment wherein the resources of the community—health, financial, and social—become the integrated for the improvement of business, families, schools, health systems, and governments.

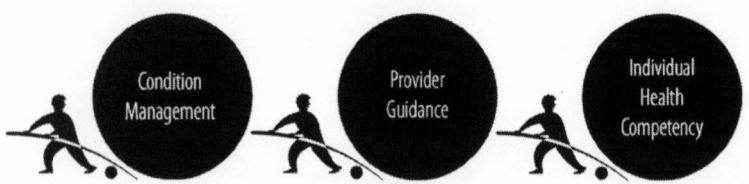

Albert Tzeel, MD, MHSA, Regional Market Medical Officer, Great Lakes Region, Humana Inc

In the book "The Ethics of the Fathers" (aka "Pirkei Avot") the great Rabbi Hillel asked three famous questions: "If I am not for myself, who is for me? When I am for myself, what am I? If not now, when?" (Chapter 1, Verse 14). One commentary on these questions promotes the concept that, rather than take these questions literally, Hillel promotes a conscious effort for the individual to balance his/her personal needs with the needs of others who comprise the greater community at large (http:// mentsh.com/avot1-14com.html). For our purposes, solving that balance is the essence of promoting individual health and healthy communities. To that end, then, it becomes incumbent upon the groups that promote and invest in health — whether they be public or private, purchasers or providers — to utilize levers of change that attain both a mindset shift and a behavioral adjustment leading an individual to meet his/her personal health needs. Why is this important? Because, as one meets his/her personal health needs, the community meets its own needs as well.

10.4 Final Thoughts

Innovative ideas can be learned and tested by any who grasp the significance. If your data shows risk that can be modified, if your designs can be improved in order to support the behavior change that you are seeking, and if you carefully watch the behavior changes to see if they are occurring in the timeline that you imagined or if they are developing unintended consequences, then you are on your way to the dividends that come from benefits designs using levers to improve outcomes.

As you build your competency, you will become more innovative. The first step in innovation is to feel secure enough that you are willing to think differently and apply skills to solve the problems differently. It's a matter of learn, do, share.

Remember that you can move through the four-step process with your consultants, your internal teams across your business, your health plan/pharmacy/condition management companies, and other business leaders in your community. Follow the four-step process of Data, Design, Delivery and Dividend.

DATA: Accumulate all the data you can from claims, disability and absenteeism, workers compensation and safety, and your service providers' book of business. Compare to the health norms in your community, if available. Then, prioritize for reducing risk and creating incentives that can deliver short-term and long-term results.

DESIGN: Use your consultants, your service providers, and other business leaders to craft alternative plan designs and augment with intermittent incentives for appropriate behaviors. Write down the goals you will achieve and how you will measure them.

DELIVERY: Consider innovations from research, from business coalitions, and from other organizations. Embed ongoing messages that are relevant to the populations you are influencing, and link the messages to business goals, community goals, and economic goals.

DIVIDENDS: Measure, refine, implement anew. Keep re-investing to drive productivity, reduce waste and risk, and teach competency. Use some of the dividends for impromptu rewards, celebrations. Be sure to communicate the success with internal management teams as well as external "stakeholders," such as family members.

Map the inputs on spreadsheets, graphs, or databases that will show you what you are doing well and where there is room for improvement. Test the ideas in small steps with early wins. Use your intuition and back it with numbers and research. Be brave and bold in your approach. And at all times, ask your employees and their families what is important to them.

At some point, we're all innovators. When you achieve success, share it with another so that more innovation will drive healthier people, healthier communities, and healthier financial outcomes.

ENDNOTES

1 http://www.kff.org/pullingittogether/041609_altman.cfm
4/17/2009

2 http://www.kff.org/insurance/upload/7670_02.pdf
accessed 3.19.09

3 Ibid.

4 Brook, R.H., "Health, Health Insurance, and the Uninsured,"
JAMA 265 (20):2998-3002, 1991

5 Goldman, D. JAMA 2004:291;2344-2350

6 Brook, R.H. op.cit.

7 http://dictionary.reference.com/browse/lever accessed 6.7.09

8 Nayer C and Mahoney JJ. Health Value Continuum. Center
for Health Value Innovation 2007

9 Center for Health Value Innovation 2007

10 Center for Health Value Innovation 2009

11 Berger, J. Managed Healthcare Executive, http://managed
health careexecutive.modernmedicine.com/mhe/article/article
Detail.jsp?id=155752 5.7.09

12 Riedel et al. J Occup Environ Med. 2009;51:283–295

13 Holben, Robert. The Gulfstream Story on Healthcare Costs
and Wellness – a Quality Journey. Excerpted from a white
paper submission to the Center for Health Transformation
2008.

14 Mahoney, JJ. Center for Health Value Innovation 2007-2009
presentations

15 Health Affairs. 1999; Vol 18, Number 5; 193-203

[16] Mahoney, JJ. "Reducing Patient Drug Acquisition Costs Can Lower Diabetes Health Claims," Am J Manag Care. 2005;11:S170-S176

[17] Cranor CW et al. J Am Pharm Assoc. 2003;43:173-184

[18] Lamphier, Roy. Detroit Chamber of Commerce, Presentation, Feb 2009

[19] Nayer, C. "Evidence to Drive Health Value," Center for Health Value Innovation, Presentation, Feb 2009

[20] http://www.nytimes.com/2009/04/23/business/23cigna.html?_r=1

[21] Nayer, C. 101 Lifetips for Personal Health Management, 2009

13160085R00087

Made in the USA
Charleston, SC
20 June 2012